KT-528-928

# Measurement Scales Used in Elderly Care

ABHAYA GUPTA MD, MRCPI

Consultant Physician
Department of Medicine and Elderly Care
West Wales Hospital
Carmarthen

*Forewords by*

JEREMY PLAYFER MD, FRCP
Consultant Geriatrician (Emeritus), Royal Liverpool University Hospital
Past President, British Geriatrics Society

and

BIM BHOWMICK OBE, MD, FRCP
Consultant Physician, Torfaen Intermediate Care
Ex-Associate Postgraduate Dean, County Hospital, Pontypool

Radcliffe Publishing
Oxford • New York

**Radcliffe Publishing Ltd**
18 Marcham Road
Abingdon
Oxon OX14 1AA
United Kingdom

**www.radcliffe-oxford.com**
Electronic catalogue and worldwide online ordering facility.

© 2008 Abhaya Gupta

Abhaya Gupta has asserted his right under the Copyright, Designs and Patents Act 1998 to be identified as the author of this work.

All rights reserved. No part of this publication may be reproduced, stored in a retrieval system or transmitted, in any form or by any means, electronic, mechanical, photocopying, recording or otherwise, without the prior permission of the copyright owner.

British Library Cataloguing in Publication Data

A catalogue record for this book is available from the British Library.

ISBN-13: 978 184619 266 1

Typeset by Pindar NZ (Egan Reid), Auckland, New Zealand
Printed and bound by TJI Digital, Padstow, Cornwall, UK

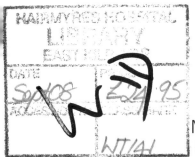

HAIRMYRES HOSPITAL
LIBRARY
EAST KILBRIDE

DATE
Sep '08

2.24.95

WT/141

369 0109185

# Measurement Scales
# Used in Elderly Care

# Contents

# Foreword

I am delighted to write this Foreword to Dr Gupta's excellent book *Measurement Scales Used in Elderly Care*. The book is clearly written and it is a much needed and scholarly addition to the geriatric canon.

Assessment is central to the practice of geriatric medicine, and Dr Gupta's introduction to and compilation of measurement scales that are useful in the practice of geriatric medicine indicate the growing maturity of the specialty. The early pioneers of the specialty used intuitive assessments based on observation and experience. However, holistic impressions are highly subjective and open to bias. The need for objectivity, based on scientifically valid and precise methodology, is obvious. Over the last 30 years much excellent research, often unrecognised, has been undertaken in the development of measurement scales for use in clinical practice. These have proved invaluable in research and audit, and as an integral part of day-to-day practice.

All members of the multi-disciplinary team working in geriatric units require a sound knowledge of the basic principles of measurement scales. We need to be competent in the use and selection of appropriate scales, and understand which scales are valid and fit for purpose. Unfortunately, up until now this has been a difficult task, often requiring reference to original papers. Dr Gupta's scholarship has now come to the rescue. He provides a critical commentary on the principles and application of clinical scales that are relevant to the management of older people. He has trawled through the many hundreds of scales available, selecting those that are most useful for the specialty.

This book will be valuable to all members of the multi-disciplinary team. It will be particularly helpful to trainees, as this knowledge is not well represented in standard textbooks and, although included in the curriculum, it is rarely taught.

The dream of a comprehensive geriatric assessment which is also objective, giving the same results when applied in different settings, has been the Holy Grail of academic geriatrics. Better information technology enables us to integrate scientifically valid rating scales within everyday practice. Serial measures allow us to track progress or recognise failure of interventions, thereby validating our practice. Comparison of the results obtained in different units facilitates both research and audit, thus benefiting patient care. There is an untapped potential for large-scale research within the specialty, given the large number of patients who pass through our units. The collection of reliable data based on measurement scales allows improved healthcare planning and management.

Dr Gupta has done an excellent job of outlining the theory and practice of measurement scales. He has put together an extremely useful compendium of scales. I congratulate him and wish his publication every success. I can foresee this publication becoming an essential text for every unit library, as well as a valuable book for individual clinicians.

**Dr Jeremy Playfer** MD, FRCP
**Consultant Geriatrician (Emeritus), Royal Liverpool University
Hospital
Past President, British Geriatrics Society**
*February 2008*

# Foreword

I am delighted to write a Foreword for this book. There is an increasing ageing population, and people with chronic disabilities are living longer thanks to improved knowledge and technology and major new developments. Effective use of appropriate resources which are in short supply is a major issue in the NHS.

The central key to multi-pathology-laden elderly people is accurate diagnosis and assessment and targeted management measures. One holistic assessment encompasses evaluation of mental, physical and social circumstances. Assessment can occur in different settings – in primary care, in the community and in hospital.

A vast number of assessment scales are available to multi-professional groups, and they are used both to grade disabilities and to monitor progress and therapeutic intervention and outcome. They are also used in research and audit.

Doctors are least knowledgeable about the assessment scales which are traditionally not taught in medical schools. Postgraduate trainees do not use these often, and have very little interest in them, as they do not form part of the core curriculum or the syllabus for higher examinations.

This book summarises the most commonly used validated assessment scales, which can be utilised by medical students, postgraduate trainees, consultants and members of the multi-disciplinary team.

I hope that a copy of this book will be kept in every ward, outpatient department and GP practice for daily use and reference.

**Professor Bim Bhowmick** OBE, MD, FRCP
**Consultant Physician, Torfaen Intermediate Care**
**Ex-Associate Postgraduate Dean**
*February 2008*

# Preface

A huge range of measurement scales have been used in medical practice, especially in geriatric medicine. Moreover, new measures are constantly being developed.

Although several larger textbooks are available, these are mainly useful for researchers, and I realised that there was a need for a handy book for use by a busy clinician. In my experience, many practitioners are overwhelmed by the number of books available on measurement scales. Here I have included some of the commonly used scales in clinical practice. This book would be useful not only for junior doctors entering training in geriatric medicine, but also for consultant geriatricians and members of the multi-disciplinary team. In this book, the emphasis is on published and clinically useful measures which are commonly utilised in geriatric practice in the UK. The book will have a valuable role in training in the elements and application of systematic assessments for doctors, nurses, administrators and social workers who work with older people.

The literature refers to hundreds of measurement scales. Some of these are of historical interest only and have not stood the test of time. Many have been adapted and modified to clinical practice as deemed appropriate. Only a few selected measures have been included in this book. Section 1 deals with the basic principles of reliable and valid scales, while Section 2 describes the actual instruments and includes copies of these wherever possible. Most of the included scales have good evidence of validity and reliability and would enhance the efficiency and effectiveness of geriatric practice. This will be an extremely valuable and practical book for busy practitioners who, due to time constraints, are unable to refer to larger textbooks and to journals. The focus is mainly on those scales which are available in English, which can be completed easily and that are in common usage. The majority of these can be used without any specialist training. Important references have been included at the end of each description of a scale. A 'Further reading' list of important textbooks for further information is also provided at the end of the book.

Some scales have been excluded because they are subject to tight copyright or are only available from original sources. Every effort has been made to seek permission from copyright holders to reproduce the scales that are included. Users of scales should be aware that the latter should not be reproduced or sold for profit, and permission to use the scales should be obtained from their original source. The scales reproduced here are not sanctioned for use elsewhere.

Finally, I would like to thank the various authors and publishers who agreed to the inclusion of their scales in this book. If copyright permissions error is discovered, I would ask the copyright holders to contact me via the publishers so that things could be put right.

**Abhaya Gupta**
*February 2008*

# About the author

**Dr Abhaya Gupta** is working as a Consultant Physician at the West Wales Hospital in Carmarthen, UK, developing local elderly care services. His special interests include stroke and osteoporosis, and he has published widely, including research articles, review articles and case reports in several journals. He is a reviewer for *Brain* and *Age and Ageing*, a member of the editorial board for *Geriatric Medicine* and *Welsh Stroke Bulletin*, and has contributed many posters and presentations at international conferences. He is a member of the British Geriatric Society, the British Association of Stroke Physicians, the Wales Osteoporosis Advisory Group and the Wales Orthogeriatric Group.

# Acknowledgements

I am indebted to my colleagues for their influence, guidance and practical advice. In addition, I wish to express my thanks to all those individuals who gave copyright permission to reproduce the scales. I would also like to thank my family for allowing me the space and time to write the book, my hospital secretary for secretarial assistance, and the hospital library staff who helped me in collecting information.

*Dedicated to the memory of my dear father,*
*Dr Rajendra Gupta, who died on 11 December 2004.*

# Introduction

A variety of assessment scales have been devised for use with elderly people. The tools have been designed to provide objective measurement of function for screening, evaluating baseline status, monitoring changes over time, determining the effects of interventions, and predicting and documenting outcomes of individuals and populations. However, the vast majority of the instruments now available were initially developed for research purposes. Many of these scales are impractical for use in clinical medicine because of their length, complexity or equipment requirements, or because they were not targeted towards older populations. However, some of them are used in clinical practice, where they have been found to be quite useful. In the following sections, some of the more commonly used assessment scales are described. These measurement scales would be useful for clinicians and other healthcare professionals who work with elderly people.

Elderly people have complex clinical presentations and needs, which necessitate a special approach to their evaluation and care. A comprehensive geriatric assessment can determine a frail elderly person's medical, psychosocial and functional capabilities. The process of comprehensive geriatric assessment is multi-dimensional – that is, in addition to medical diagnostic evaluation, it determines functional status and quality of life through frequent use of standardised measurement instruments. In the elderly population, a holistic assessment and use of assessment scales form part of a holistic approach. This is essential to describe the many ways in which the disease interacts to cause impairment, disability and handicap. Use of scales is invaluable as a means of reducing uncertainty in diagnosis, monitoring and evaluating prognosis. The scales can be considered as a technology of healthcare for elderly people, which clearly needs to be simple, user-friendly and applicable across a wide range of settings and professions. In the UK, the Royal College of Physicians and the British Geriatrics Society recommend the use of assessment scales as part of standard clinical practice in recording the health status of elderly people.

Health professionals working with elderly people in primary or secondary care should incorporate some of these tools into their clinical practice. Service managers will need these instruments for service development. Researchers use them to increase our knowledge about conditions that affect the elderly.

1

# Section 1

## DEFINITION OF SCALES

A scale is a series of question, ratings or items that is used to measure a concept. The response categories are then summed and statistical calculations can be performed on the summed scores. In other words, scales are numerical values that are used to represent attributes of quantities, qualities or categories The measurement scales are expected to be explicit and unambiguous, thereby implying an ability to standardise the concept. However, there are several practical considerations that must be taken into account when deciding which is the appropriate tool to use in a particular situation. Several measurement scales are available in the medical literature which are a means of identifying groups or individuals who have or will develop some target condition or outcome.

## THE NEED FOR ASSESSMENT SCALES

### Assessment of the older person

*Assessment* is defined as the process of objectively defining the needs of a person. This is to enable them to achieve, maintain or restore an acceptable level of social independence or quality of life. The scales help to achieve these needs, which may be simple or comprehensive.

The assessment of an older person is a complex process. Such assessments are needed in a variety of different settings – in primary care, in the hospital and in long-stay homes. Assessment scales for the elderly are necessary to enable an accurate diagnosis to be made, progress to be monitored and outcome to be evaluated. Such scales can measure different aspects of a person's health and well-being – physical, mental and/or social. In some cases the diagnosis may be missed unless scales are used. Assessment scales also provide a baseline for making treatment decisions. Standardised scales are a useful tool in comprehensive assessment of older people prior to entry to long-term care. In addition, scales are available to measure the needs of the carers, their home conditions and their social status. The instruments provide a baseline measurement and can be repeated when progress needs to be monitored. The measurements quantify the extent of a problem. They permit tabulation of clinical data and enable measurement of changes over time. They are the means by which problems and goals are defined and the achievement of goals is gauged. They are useful for evaluating outcomes by monitoring changes in health status of the individual. They can also be used to evaluate the effectiveness of an intervention. They establish a degree of uniformity in clinical assessment. Thus the scales enable comprehensive geriatric assessment to be more reliable, and they ensure consistency in the assessment process. In the hospital setting in particular, in acute care, but also in rehabilitation and long-term care of the elderly, these scales can be used to collect information that aids diagnosis, treatment and determination of the prognosis.

In general, there are three main ways to measure outcomes in the older patient:
1  a change in a particular scale or scales
2  measurement of the end points of a disease, admission to hospital, length of hospital stay or institutionalisation
3  death.

The NHS and Community Care Act proposals state that some form of assessment is necessary to ensure delivery of appropriate support and resources to disabled elderly people in the community.[1] The use of assessment scales is not simply a matter of 'ticking boxes', but provides a commitment to a holistic approach in which geriatric medicine has supremacy over any other branch of medicine. Since describing disabilities is one of the key aspects of management of elderly patients, use of standardised scales could enhance clinical care.

## Communication between healthcare professionals and researchers

The scales aid communication of clinically relevant quantitative information among different healthcare professionals. They encourage the development of a common clinical knowledge, thereby aiding communication, especially in hospital practice, where so many professionals are involved both in multi-disciplinary teams and with external agencies. Thus they enhance clinical care in geriatric medical practice.

## Audit

The scales are helpful in clinical audit of conditions that are prevalent in older people. Audit of service by the use of assessment scales could indicate whether or not the service is effective. These scales enable more meaningful comparisons to be made between clinicians, units or districts. This could enhance the quality of care, and is also useful in service evaluation and development.

## Screening of disease and disability

Standardised scales are useful in screening of disability, impairment and handicap both in primary care (e.g. 'over-75' health checks) and in hospital settings. In this way various population norms have been produced (e.g. the prevalence of dementia in the population). The Office of Population Censuses and Surveys scales have been used to study the extent of disability in the population in the

UK. The elderly screening initiative can identify a high prevalence of unreported physical, social and psychological needs of the elderly living in the community.

## Health planning and management

Assessment scales can provide valuable information on the prevalence of disability, cognitive impairment and social well-being both during hospital contacts and in the community. Scales are helpful in planning services and determining allocation of appropriate resources by health and social services. They are the means by which resources needed for adequate healthcare for the elderly can be weighed against other competing demands. For example, the need for services for disabled people in the community can be determined. Assessment scales support clinical and service management in medical practice. With the rapidly changing organisational reforms in the NHS in the UK, the availability of standardised information on patient well-being can meet many of the management objectives.

## Research

Assessment scales are very useful in clinical, epidemiological and health services research concerning elderly people. Interface with research occurs particularly when a clinician evaluates gerontological literature in which measurements are used to study the effects of clinical treatment or management interventions on the functioning and health of the patient. Indeed some geriatricians will be using these scales for their clinical research as well.

## WHICH SCALE SHOULD BE USED?

In view of the wide variety of scales available, an important decision faced by the professional is which scale to apply. Several scales are available for measuring the various symptoms, conditions and diseases in older people. Some of them have been used more often than others, and have been tested repeatedly. Healthcare professionals must be confident both that they are choosing instruments which are appropriate for their clients, and that they are administering and interpreting those instruments correctly.

The elderly suffer a variety of chronic diseases (e.g. stroke, heart disease, arthritis) that accumulate over the lifespan, and certain *disease-specific scales* have been designed to assess a particular disease. Moreover, functional ability, mental health, social status and quality of life are also essential elements of the health of an older person, and these can be measured by *generic scales*. Thus measurements in older people require a multi-dimensional approach in which the following are assessed individually:

- physical health – disease-specific measures
- mental health:
  - cognitive functioning
  - mood (anxiety, depression)
- functional status – functional capability
- social status – includes broader aspects of health (life satisfaction, morale, social support).

The multi-dimensional tools usually assess a variety of medical, social, physical or emotional domains and provide a summary score of the overall result. They are most useful in survey research because of the need to collect a large amount of information at one time. However, in a clinical setting, healthcare professionals would choose instruments that focus on a specific area of interest.

There are many scales available from which to choose, and there is no consensus on which package should be used in different settings. Several issues need to be considered when selecting an assessment scale for a specific population. When choosing a measurement, the most important consideration is why it is being used. The commonest reason for undertaking a measurement is to ascertain the diagnosis, prognosis, severity and outcome of a condition. Discriminative tools are used to distinguish individuals who have a particular problem from those who do not (e.g. the Berg Scale is useful for identifying fall-prone elderly people in the community). Similarly, an evaluative tool is used to measure change over time or after treatment (e.g. the Modified Rankin Scale). Scale validity, reliability (discussed later), patient acceptance, time and personnel needed to administer the instrument, and the relevance and usefulness of the data to be collected are important considerations. Scale simplicity is also important, as an instrument may not be suitable for routine use if it is too long or requires highly trained interviewers. A simple test can improve patient and user compliance, and is quicker and easier to use. If the quantitative assessment is simple, it is relatively easy for both clinician and patient. The amount of time available, space, equipment and staff training are resource-related factors that need to be considered. It should be remembered that limiting the number of variables in a scale contributes to simplicity and utility but may result in loss of completeness and sensitivity. Its purpose in relation to the characteristics of the population used is also relevant, as instruments used in one context may be unsuitable in another. The scale should be well designed and in an appropriate format and language for both the subjects and the different users of that scale. It must fit into the pattern of routine clinical practice. Another important feature is communicability – it should be possible to communicate the results to others without difficulty. It is best to use an existing scale which is appropriate to the needs of the population that is being tested. This avoids the need to establish the validity and reliability of the scale, and in addition the scale will be familiar to other users. Thus both methodological and practical issues should guide the choice of an instrument.

---

**SUMMARY CHECKLIST TO BE COMPLETED BEFORE USING A SCALE**

- Is the scale appropriate for the purpose?
- To what extent is the scale valid, reliable, sensitive and specific?
- Who is administering the scale?
- Who is the scale intended for?
- Can a proxy respondent complete it?
- How long does it take to administer the scale?
- What is the acceptability of the scale to both patient and user?
- How is the questionnaire scored?
- Are the scores weighted?
- Are the scores skewed (ceiling or floor effects)?
- Can the results be readily communicated to others?

---

In the following sections some of the scales commonly used in geriatric practice in the UK are discussed. The instruments described in detail are some of the most widely used and best validated tools in clinical use. Wherever possible, the scales have been reproduced in full. Either one scale or a combination of scales can be used, depending upon the questions that need to be answered and the individual circumstances. Exclusion of any particular scale from this book does not reflect negatively on that scale. The Royal College of Physicians and the British Geriatrics Society joint workshop has examined assessment scales for the elderly and recommended some of the most useful instruments.[2]

## SOME USEFUL PROPERTIES OF SCALES

### Reliability

Reliability is the ability of a scale to produce consistent results on a number of different occasions. In other words, it is the ability to obtain the same result with repeated measurements. Reliability includes both reproducibility among observers and consistency among scale items. It is important because the error is increased if there is poor reproducibility over consecutive tests or among different observers.

Observer reliability is best assessed with the k-statistic, which is a measure of agreement developed for the study of non-parametric ratings by observers,[3] and is defined as follows:

$$k = \frac{(Po - Pe)}{(1 - Pe)}$$

where Po is the observed proportion of agreement and Pe is the proportion of agreement expected by chance.[3]

Thus k accounts for agreement expected on the basis of chance. Reliability ranges from −1 for complete disagreement to +1 for perfect agreement. The degree of assessment is conventionally interpreted as < 0 = poor, 0–0.2 = slight, 0.21–0.40 = fair, 0.41–0.60 = moderate, 0.61–0.80 = substantial and 0.81–1.0 = almost perfect. Weighted k-statistics are useful for scale items that contain more than two possible responses in order to more accurately reflect the inter-observer agreement.

Reliability can be judged in the following ways:
- *Test-retest reliability* is the ability to achieve consistent results following administration of the scale on different occasions to the same population (i.e. consistency over time). Potential problems are include the possibility that first administration could affect the second response, observation error, and genuine individual change error.
- *Internal consistency* is the measurement of the same concept by different scale items (i.e. the extent to which all of the items measure the same dimension). Basic tests include split half, item–item correlations and item–total correlations. It involves testing for homogeneity. Internal consistency is calculated by using the KR20 formula developed by Kuder–Richardson for items with only two possible responses, or Cronbach's alpha coefficient for items with more than two possible responses.[4] Cronbach's alpha coefficient is a coefficient of correlation with values ranging from 0 to 1. An alpha coefficient of > 0.8 is considered to be good, and of > 0.9 is considered to be excellent. Thus higher values indicate better consistency.[4]
- *Inter-rater reliability* is the consistency of a measure when administered by different interviewers on a single occasion. This can be improved by intensive training of individuals using scales.
- *Intra-rater reliability* is the reliability of measurement by the same rater of the same subjects on different occasions (repeat testing). The elderly show fluctuations in their mental and functional abilities, so it is important to distinguish between a change in score resulting from real change and one that is due to some artefact.
- *Sensitivity to change* is the instrument's responsiveness to change with the

change in clinical condition. This would involve correlation with other measures (e.g. a depression scale would need to correlate with a structured psychiatric interview for any changes in psychological status).

## Validity

Validity is the extent to which a scale accurately measures the underlying concept – that is, whether the measure chosen achieves its intended purpose. There are several aspects of validity.

- *Criterion validity* is the extent to which the measure correlates with a 'gold standard.' This situation can occur when a new measurement is being developed as a single alternative to an existing one. Criterion validity is subdivided into *concurrent validity* and *predictive validity*, depending on whether the criterion refers to the current or future state.
- *Content validity*. Does the scale include all of the relevant concepts that are due to be measured? A multi–item scale should include all aspects of its content. Content validation relies on expert opinions and reviews of the literature (e.g. National Institutes of Health Stroke Scale items were selected on the basis of previously studied scales and experience of investigators).
- *Construct validity* is demonstrated by examining the relationships between a newly created test and other tests to show that the new test measures the same 'construct.' This is most useful when a definite criterion for comparison (i.e. 'gold standard') does not exist, as for example in the measurement of intelligence or anxiety. Observable phenomena such as weakness, sensory loss, aphasia, etc. in stroke provide information about a single underlying 'construct.'
- *Face validity*. Is the scale appropriate on face value?
- *Discriminant validity*. Does the scale distinguish patients who are deemed to be different?

Validity is often more difficult to assess. Moreover, validity is not an absolute property of a scale but a relative one. For example, a scale could be valid for one purpose but invalid for other purposes.

## Responsiveness to change

This is the ability of an instrument to detect change, especially clinically important changes. A scale should be capable of detecting a change related to time or interventions at all levels of the scale. It may not be able to detect meaningful differences between subjects who score near the bottom or top of the scale (these are referred to as 'floor' and 'ceiling' effects, respectively).

## Sensitivity and specificity

The scale should categorise people accurately, especially when used for screening.

▶ *Sensitivity* is the percentage of true positives (TP) – that is, avoiding false negatives (FN). Sensitivity is an indication of how well a test identifies people who truly have the condition of interest. It is calculated using the following equation:

$$\text{Sensitivity} = TP/(TP+FN).$$

- *True positives* are people who test positively for a particular condition and actually have that condition.
- *False negatives* are people who test negatively for a particular condition but actually have that condition.

▶ *Specificity* is the number of true negatives (TN) as a percentage of all negatives – that is, avoiding false positives (FP). Sensitivity is an indication of how well a test identifies people who truly do not have the condition of interest. It is calculated using the following equation:

$$\text{Specificity} = TN/(FP+TN).$$

- *True negatives* are people who test negatively for a particular condition and actually do not have that condition.
- *False positives* are people who test positively for a particular condition but actually do not have that condition.

Any instrument can yield false-positive or false-negative results. The absolute number of false-positive or false-negative results will depend upon the likelihood of the phenomenon being present in the population being tested.

An instrument that is to be used for screening must have high sensitivity and specificity. No instrument is perfect, so there must be a trade-off between sensitivity and specificity. Raising the cut-off point to reduce false-positive results will improve specificity but may increase false-negative results and therefore result in a decrease in sensitivity. The acceptable levels of sensitivity and specificity will depend upon the nature of the disease. The levels of sensitivity and specificity could vary depending upon their context of use. For example, the Mini Mental State Examination (MMSE) has falsely high positive rates for poorly educated people and falsely high negative rates for well-educated people.

The relationship between true and false positive can also be expressed by *positive predictive value (PPV)*. This is the proportion of all instrument positives that are true positives – in other words, how likely it is that a positive result from a test indicates the presence of a real disease. This concept is important in interpreting screening results. The PPV is sensitive to the prevalence of the condition that is being screened for, such that the greater the prevalence, the higher the PPV.

## Weighting scale scoring

Scales can be criticised with regard to the method of attributing equal weights to item responses. For example, with responses per item ranging from 1 to 20, the higher the score the less the disability, but it cannot be assumed that 20 is 20 times as bad as 1. Moreover, many scales give each item an equal scoring weight. Although this is an easy solution, some items could be more important than others. Furthermore, a given score could be reached in different ways. For example, a cheerful and lucid patient who is unable to walk due to arthritis could have the same scale score as a person who is physically mobile but disorientated.

## Precision of an item response

The finer the distinction that can be made between the subject's responses, the greater the precision of the scale. For example, asking a person to simply agree or disagree with a statement yields only two possible responses (this is known as a *dichotomous* response). Respondents could be asked for their opinion along a continuum – for example, 'strongly disagree, disagree, no opinion, agree or strongly agree' (Likert scale).[5] This is relevant for scales that address attitudinal and behavioural issues. The continuum should not be too great, otherwise meaningless responses could be elicited. One approach could be to indicate replies on a visual analogue scale on a line corresponding to the respondent's state. Alternatively, these visual analogue rating scales can measure chronic or temporary health states. A typical rating scale consists of a line drawn on a page with clear end points (e.g. 'death' at one end and 'healthy' at the other). The respondent's health status is then located on a line between these two end points. Scale measurements are rated from 0 (worst) to 1 (best). Another example is the Visual Analogue Pain Scale. A range of other response scales have been described.[6] The choice of response format also determines the type of statistics which can be applied.

## WHO SHOULD PERFORM THE ASSESSMENT?

There is some debate as to who is the best person to use these scales in the elderly. The majority of assessments are made by the clinician (e.g. general practitioner, hospital doctor, geriatrician) or by a therapist (e.g. occupational therapist), and some are made by a practice nurse or a health visitor. However, any individual with well-developed interviewing and communication skills, knowledge about care of the elderly and a positive attitude towards ageing may use these scales. The relative involvement of health and social care agencies in performing various assessments varies. However, in view of the multi-agency involvement in elderly care, duplication between agencies and over-assessment need to be avoided. A joint agreement policy for use of assessment methods can ensure that 'seamless care' is provided. At local levels, mechanisms should be developed to ensure quality of care in the community for elderly people by establishing closer working relationships among the key personnel involved.

The scales that are used are broadly of three types.

### Self-completion scales

These are completed by the respondent him- or herself. Postal questionnaires have the following advantages.

▶ They are time saving, as questions can be sent by post/answered at the clinic.
▶ Larger samples can be used.
▶ They are useful in any setting.
▶ They reduce staffing and resources costs.
▶ They are useful for follow-up.

The respondent may be:

▶ a patient/subject
▶ a third party (e.g. partner or other relative, nurse, care worker)
▶ a relative or friend who helps the patient with the answers.

### Interviewer-administered questionnaires

These have the following advantages.

▶ This personal approach maximises responses and yields a higher response rate.
▶ More valid results are obtained, as difficulties can be clarified by the interviewers.
▶ This approach is especially helpful in the elderly in the initial stages, when the cognitive state and educational level of the subject are not known.
▶ More information can be collected with open-ended questions.
▶ More sensitive and complex issues can be discussed.

Their disadvantages are as follows.

▶ A clinician or researcher must be present.
▶ The approach is restricted with regard to geographical area.
▶ Interviewer skills are important, so training may be needed.

## Equipment-based evaluations

These could provide more objective and responsive measures of functional performance than self-reports or interviewer-administered questionnaires. However, they are usually more expensive than the other formats, due to the costs associated with purchase and upkeep of the necessary equipment. Moreover, unless the equipment can be easily transported, the individual who is to be assessed must come to the facility where the equipment is housed.

## WHAT IS BEING MEASURED? DOMAINS OF ASSESSMENT SCALES

Assessment instruments in the elderly cover a wide range of areas relevant to the health and well-being of elderly people. The main areas of interest and some useful instruments are mentioned below. The Royal College of Physicians/ British Geriatrics Society joint workshop in 1992 identified seven domains for the assessment of elderly people:[2]

1 physical health
2 mental health
3 activities of daily living
4 psychosocial functioning
5 social resources
6 economic resources
7 environmental resources.

In clinical practice, there are five main areas to assess an elderly person's health. They are: physical health, functional ability, mental health, quality of life, and carer strain.

## Physical health or disease

Most clinicians quantify physical health or disease by compiling a problem list of defined diagnoses and symptom complexes. Documenting the number of days of hospitalisation and using the New York Heart Association Dyspnoea Scale are the common examples. However, a number of detailed, disease-specific scales are available. Some of these are purely quantitative, some are qualitative (e.g. including quality-of-life issues), while others include both aspects.

Examples of disease-specific scales include the following:
▶ the Hoehn and Yahr Scale and the Webster Scale for parkinsonism
▶ the National Institutes of Health Stroke Scale, the Scandinavian Stroke Scale and the Canadian Stroke Scale for stroke.

## Functional ability

In the elderly, measurement of functional ability is an essential part of clinical practice. The major domains of functional ability include *activities of daily living (ADL)* and *instrumental activities of daily living (IADL)*. ADL are basic physical self-care activities that a person must be able to perform in order to survive without help. They include eating, dressing, transferring, toileting and bathing. IADL are an extension of ADL, and include more complex tasks such as heavy housework, cooking, shopping, laundry, taking medication, managing finances and using the telephone. These are activities that a person must be able to perform in order to remain independent without outside help. ADL are disability oriented, whereas IADL assess handicap rather than disability.

More than 100 ADL scales have been described in the literature. Examples of functional ability scales include the following:

▶ the Barthel Index
▶ the Katz ADL scale
▶ the Lawton ADL scale
▶ the PULSES Profile
▶ the Northwick Park ADL scale
▶ the Functional Independence Measure (FIM)
▶ the Frenchay Activities Index.

These functional scales help health professionals to detect problems in performing daily activities, and to determine the type of assistance needed by the person who is being assessed. Impairment of basic activities indicates that caregiver or nursing home support is needed for survival.

## Mental health

This is an important part of the assessment of patients with dementia. However, the role of scales is not confined to the diagnosis of dementia. They are used to assess the cognitive ability of older people as well as their behavioural competence. Measurement of mental health and well-being includes three major categories. These are commonly used across specialties of psychiatry, geriatrics and neurology.

### Cognition (mental status)

The tests of cognition include:

▶ the Abbreviated Mental Test (AMT)
▶ the Mini Mental State Examination (MMSE)
▶ the Clifton Assessment Procedures for the Elderly (CAPE).

### Affect (anxiety and depression)

The tests of affect include:
- the Hospital Anxiety and Depression Scale
- the Yesavage Geriatric Depression Scale
- the Hamilton Depression Rating Scale
- the Zung Self-Rating Depression Scale.

### Behaviour

The tests of behaviour include:
- the Clifton Assessment Procedures for the Elderly (CAPE)
- the Behavioural Pathology in Alzheimer's Disease (BEHAVE-AD) Rating Scale
- the Manchester and Oxford Universities Scales for Psychopathological Assessment of Dementia (MOUSEPAD).

## Quality-of-life assessment

An important aspect of clinical practice is to understand and measure changes in patients' well-being. Well-being is part of a broader concept, namely *quality of life (QOL)*, which is defined as encompassing all aspects of human life – material and physical components, social, emotional and spiritual well-being. In the absence of disease, QOL is a personal and variable concept that means different things to different people. Parameters that are useful in assessing QOL include home and family situation, satisfaction with life, health status, presence and severity of suffering, employment and availability of health services. All of these have an impact on QOL. A global measurement of change in a person's QOL before and after intervention has become increasingly popular in drug trials. QOL scales identify the overall health behaviour of the population. They are not useful for screening. A good QOL instrument for use should have the following three main properties:
- It should be easy to use (i.e. it should contain short questions, with clear instructions).
- It should be easy for patients to understand, and should not cause distress.
- It should have the capacity to detect change.

Examples of QOL scales include the following:
- the Short Form 36 (SF-36)
- the Nottingham Health Profile
- the Sickness Impact Profile
- the Philadelphia Geriatric Center Morale scale.

*Quality-adjusted-life years (QALYs)* have been proposed as a measure of the health index of the population. This is helpful in resource allocation.

## Carer strain

Elderly people in the community are dependent upon the help and support provided by families and carers. Most carers are women, they are often elderly themselves, and they provide care over long periods for chronically disabled people. Assessment instruments have been devised to monitor the level of burden and stress on carers. Carer burden is a broad term that includes deterioration in the physical and mental health of the carer, financial difficulties and disruption of family life.

Examples of carer scales which have been used in the elderly include the following:

▶ the Caregiver Strain Index
▶ the Relatives' Stress Score.

### IN WHAT SETTINGS SHOULD THE SCALE BE USED?

The measurement scales could be applicable in a variety of settings, as listed below.

▶ *Rehabilitation wards.* Scales that assess the functional status of patients can document progress, and are used in specialised rehabilitation settings.
▶ *Geriatric units.* Scales that assess frail elderly subjects are useful for determining diagnosis and prognosis and for monitoring in either acute or long-stay facilities.
▶ *Community-dwelling elderly.* Physical and mental health has been studied in several elderly populations across the world. Subjective well-being of the population can be determined. Various community norms have been produced (e.g. prevalence of dementia).
▶ *Psychogeriatric units.* This could include both inpatient and outpatient services.

### REFERENCES

1 Office of Public Sector Information. *NHS and Community Care Act 1990.* London: HMSO; 1990.
2 Royal College of Physicians of London and the British Geriatrics Society. *Standardised Assessment Scales for Elderly People. Report of joint workshops of the Research Unit of Royal College of Physicians of London and the British Geriatrics Society.* London: Royal College of Physicians of London; 1992.

3 Fliess JL. *Statistical Methods for Rates and Properties.* 2nd ed. New York: John Wiley & Sons Inc.; 1981.

4 Feinstein AR. *Clinimetrics.* New Haven, CT: Yale University Press; 1987.

5 Likert R. A technique for the development of attitude scales. *Educ Psychol Meas.* 1952; **12**: 313–15.

6 Bowling A. *Measuring Disease.* 2nd ed. Buckingham: Open University Press; 2001.

# Section 2

In this section, commonly used instruments that have applications in clinical practice are described.

# GLASGOW COMA SCALE

The Glasgow Coma Scale (GCS) is the scale most commonly used to assess the level of consciousness.[1] It was developed in order to assess consciousness with ease and to standardise clinical observations of patients with impaired consciousness. Before the GCS was introduced, a variety of terms, such as 'stupor' and 'semi-consciousness', were used to describe patients. The GCS assesses two aspects of consciousness:

1 arousal – awareness of the environment
2 cognition – demonstration of understanding by the ability to perform tasks.

## Scoring

This is based on three modes of behaviour:

1 best eye opening – based on a 4-point scale (from 1 to 4)
2 best verbal response – based on a 5-point scale (from 1 to 5)
3 best motor response – based on a 6-point scale (from 1 to 6).

The scores are added together to give an overall assessment of the patient's neurological status. A score of 15 represents maximum responsiveness, while a score of 3 is denotes minimum responsiveness. A score of 8 or less indicates that the patient is comatose. The following points should be noted.

▶ Due to ptosis a person may not be able to open their eyes.
▶ Best motor response is tested by the patient's ability to obey simple commands – for example, 'Put out your tongue', 'Hold up your right hand', 'Touch your right ear.' Avoid using the command 'Squeeze my fingers', as this is a primitive reflex and may occur involuntarily.
▶ Best verbal response is tested by asking the patient simple questions. Do not raise your voice. Assess whether the patient is oriented (i.e. aware of who they are (name), where they are, and the time of day (morning, evening or night). The month, year, date and day of the week are not required. Factors such as dysphasia, presence of an endotracheal/tracheostomy tube and fracture of the mandible could give falsely low results.

## Administration time

The scale takes about 2 minutes to administer.

## Validity

Since its original description, the GCS has been adapted for use as a pre-hospital triage tool for acute trauma. The aim of such a tool is to accurately identify seriously injured patients for transfer to appropriate locations for treatment. The GCS has been found to discriminate well between survivors and non-survivors.[2] At a cut-off value of ≤ 6 the sensitivity of the GCS was 87.8% and the specificity was 89.1%,[2] supporting the view that it is an effective triage tool. The GCS was also found to be an independent predictor of hospitalisation, with a lower GCS score being associated with a higher risk of hospitalisation.[3]

A number of studies have been published describing the validity of *admission GCS* as a predictor of survival after trauma. A retrospective case series of 29 000 patients in the USA identified motor response of the GCS as a highly significant and independent predictor of mortality.[4] A prospective case series demonstrated good discrimination between survivors and non-survivors, and good predictive reliability.[5]

Patients with a GCS score of < 9 were nearly 5 times more likely to be disabled at 12-month follow-up.[6]

A recent review of published studies in the literature showed that GCS scores are most accurate at predicting outcomes in head-injured patients when they are combined with patient age and papillary response, and better prediction occurs with very high or very low GCS scores.[7]

### Reliability

The value of the GCS as a trauma score and triage tool is reliant on the ease and reliability with which the scale can be applied in a variety of different situations and patient types. In their original description, Teasdale and Jennett[1] reported a high degree of consistency by different observers, but this included a small population of head-injured patients.

One study suggested a difference in the accuracy and consistency of the GCS between experienced and inexperienced staff,[8] with experienced nurses being more consistent than less experienced and student nurses. However, another study[9] showed that the GCS provides a consistent and reliable assessment irrespective of staff member status.

### Clinical applications

The GCS was first introduced in the 1970s to provide a simple and reliable method of recording and monitoring change in the level of consciousness of head-injured patients. Since then it has been widely used in trauma patients, and its use has expanded beyond its original intentions. It can be used to monitor the progress of head-injured patients, and patients with neurological and intracranial disorders, such as encephalitis, stroke and meningitis. It has also been used extensively to predict outcomes in traumatic brain-injured patients.

The GCS is simple, quick, practical and easy to use. It can be easily be administered at the bedside without the need for any equipment or special training. It can be used by doctors, nurses and paramedics. It has proved very practical in general hospital, acute trauma and neurosurgical units. It provides a quick means of evaluating acutely ill patients. In order to detect changes in consciousness, frequent scoring is needed. The GCS is sensitive to change, which is helpful when making decisions about management such as radiological imaging and neurosurgical intervention. It also allows the duration of coma to be defined more precisely in terms of how long different levels of responsiveness have persisted.

### Limitations

Although the criteria for GCS scoring are well defined, the accuracy of responses can be affected by complications such as sedation, intoxication, facial injury and endotracheal intubation. In addition, several confounding factors can affect the reliability and validity of the GCS. Verbal response is affected by hearing loss, psychiatric disorders, dementia, developmental delay, and mouth and throat injury. Motor response is affected by spinal cord and peripheral nerve injury.

---

**GLASGOW COMA SCALE**

Eye opening response
- None, 1 point
- To pain, 2 points
- To speech, 3 points
- Spontaneous, 4 points

Best motor response
- None, 1 point
- Extension, 2 points
- Abnormal flexion, 3 points
- Withdrawal, 4 points
- Localises pain, 5 points
- Obeys commands, 6 points

Best verbal response
- None, 1 point
- Incomprehensible, 2 points
- Inappropriate, 3 points
- Confused, 4 points
- Oriented, 5 points

Reproduced with the permission of Elsevier Publications from Teasdale G, Jennett B. Assessment of coma and impaired consciousness. A practical scale. *Lancet.* 1974; **2:** 81–4.

---

One study reported an inability to test the verbal response in 58% of cases, and the eye opening response could not be tested in 7% of cases, although the motor response could be assessed in all cases.[10] Without the verbal response, the total GCS score cannot be calculated. However, there is growing evidence to suggest that the motor component of the GCS alone could prove useful for predicting outcome in a trauma setting.

Thirty years after its first publication, the GCS is still used worldwide to describe and assess impaired consciousness.

## REFERENCES

1 Teasdale G, Jennett B. Assessment of coma and impaired consciousness. A practical scale. *Lancet.* 1974; **2**: 81–4.

2 Bouillon B, Lefering R, Vorweg M *et al.* Trauma score systems. Cologne validation study. *J Trauma.* 1997; **42**: 652–8.

3 Norwood SH, McAuley CE, Berne JD *et al.* A prehospital Glasgow Coma Scale score of ≤ 14 accurately predicts the need for full trauma team activation and patient hospitalisation. *J Trauma.* 2002; **53**: 503–7.

4 Meredith W, Rutledge R, Hansen A *et al.* Field triage of trauma patients based upon the ability to follow commands: a study in 29,573 injured patients. *J Trauma.* 1995; **38**: 129–35.

5 Kuhls D, Malone D, McCarter R *et al.* Predictors of mortality in adult trauma patients. *J Am Coll Surg.* 2002; **194**: 695–704.

6 Wagner A, Hammond F, Sasser H *et al.* Use of injury severity variables in determining disability and community integration after traumatic brain injury. *J Trauma.* 2000; **49**: 411–19.

7 McNett M. A review of the predictive ability of Glasgow Coma Scale scores in head-injured patients. *J Neurosci Nurs.* 2007; **39**: 68–75.

8 Rowley G, Fielding K. Reliability and accuracy of the Glasgow Coma Scale with experienced and inexperienced users. *Lancet.* 1991; **337**: 535–8.

9 Juarez J, Lyons M. Inter-rater reliability of the Glasgow Coma Scale. *J Neurosci Nurs.* 1995; **27**: 283–6.

10 Starmark J, Stalhammar D, Holmgren E *et al.* A comparison of the Glasgow Coma scale and the Reaction Level Scale. *J Neurosurg.* 1988; **69**: 699–706.

## ABBREVIATED MENTAL TEST

The Abbreviated Mental Test (AMT) is a brief test of cognitive mental function, and is one of the most commonly utilised scales in older people. It was first introduced by Hodkinson in 1972,[1] and is simple, quick and easy to use.

### Scoring

The AMT needs to be administered by an interviewer. It takes only a few minutes to complete, so is very practical to use. There are 10 questions, and each correct answer is given a score of 1. The responses are then totalled. The maximum possible score is 10. The cut-off values used by investigators have ranged from < 6 to < 10, the best cut-off value being 7. A score of < 7 suggests dementia. A score of between 8 and 10 is regarded as normal. A false low result may be caused by a sleepy patient, a distracting environment, psychoactive drugs, delirium or depression.

### Administration time

The test takes less than 5 minutes to administer.

### Reliability and validity

The test is valid against clinical assessments of dementia, and also correlates well with neuropathological changes seen at autopsy. It has been assessed in the community as well as in institutional settings, with good inter-observer reliability and repeatability.[2,3] For detection of mild dementia, correlation data suggest that the AMT is equivalent to the MMSE in a screening group (30% sensitivity and 90–96% specificity).[1] In a study of a large sample of 2808 older medical inpatients, the AMT achieved high sensitivity (81%), high specificity (84%) and a high negative predictive value (99%), but a low positive predictive value (25%). The authors of the study concluded that an AMT score of > 6 rules out dementia reliably, but that a score of < 7 requires a second level of cognitive assessment to confirm dementia.[4]

### Clinical applications

The advantage of the AMT is that it is simple to administer and score. This test has been used extensively as a simple screening tool for dementia in the community as well as hospital settings. It is almost exclusively a test of memory. If behaviour assessment is also required, the Clifton Assessment Procedure for the Elderly (CAPE) instrument can be used, which covers cognition as well as behaviour. The AMT has been recommended by the Royal College of Physicians and British

Geriatrics Society joint workshop for routine assessment of cognitive function.[5] (Note that these recommendations, published in 1992, have not been revised.)

### Limitations

The AMT has not been validated in primary care and screening populations. It is difficult to translate it either linguistically or culturally without revalidation, and several questions would need to be altered in order to update them for the twenty-first century. As this test is culturally specific, it is becoming outdated in an increasingly multi-cultural society in the UK. The AMT is not suitable for use as an outcome measure in clinical dementia trials, or for monitoring the therapeutic response to anti-dementia drugs, because it is insensitive to change. The results will be falsely low in the presence of a sleepy patient, a distracting environment or psychoactive drug effects. The AMT has been used since 1972 to aid recognition of a geriatric giant – confusion – by quantifying cognitive impairment at the bedside, but the Mini Mental State Examination (MMSE) is now being adapted for use in old age psychiatry and geriatrics.[6] One of the reasons for this is the increasing lack of relevance of the question about the 'year in which the First World War began' to the present-day population, and the substitution of 'year in which the Second World War began' has not been validated as an equivalent measure.[5] Furthermore, the AMT is considered to be a very basic and crude test of memory and/or orientation, and is not comprehensive. It is likely that this scale will be replaced by the MMSE in the future.

A shortened version, known as the AMT-7, has also been developed.[7]

---

**ABBREVIATED MENTAL TEST**

- What is your age?
- What is the time (to the nearest hour)?
- What is the year?
- What is the name of the place where you are at the moment?
- Give the patient an address (e.g. 42 West Street) for recall at the end of the test.
- Can the patient recognise two persons?
- What is your date of birth (date and month are sufficient)?
- Give the year in which the First World War began.
- Give the name of the present monarch.
- Count backwards from 20 to 1.

Reproduced with the permission of Oxford University Press from Hodkinson HM. Evaluation of a mental test score for assessment of mental impairment in the elderly. *Age Ageing.* 1972; **1**: 233–8.

---

## REFERENCES

1 Hodkinson HM. Evaluation of a mental test score for assessment of mental impairment in the elderly. *Age Ageing.* 1972; **1**: 233–8.

2 Brocklehurst JC, Carty MH, Leeming JT *et al.* Medical screening of old people accepted for residential care. *Lancet.* 1978; **ii**: 141–3.

3 Quereshi KN, Hodgkinson HM. Evaluation of a ten-question mental test in the institutionalised elderly. *Age Ageing.* 1974; **3**: 152–7.

4 Antonelli Incalzi R, Cesari M, Pedone C *et al.* Construct validity of the Abbreviated Mental Test in older medical inpatients. *Dement Geriatr Cogn Disord.* 2003; **15**: 199–206.

5 Royal College of Physicians of London and the British Geriatrics Society. *Standardised Assessment Scales for Elderly People. Report of joint workshops of the Research Unit of Royal College of Physicians of London and the British Geriatrics Society.* London: Royal College of Physicians of London; 1992.

6 Starr J, MacLullich A. Abbreviated Mental Test. *Br Geriatr Soc Newsletter.* 2006; **May issue**: 3.

7 Jitapunkul S, Pillay I, Ebrahim S. The Abbreviated Mental Test. *Age Ageing.* 1991; **20**: 332–6.

## MINI MENTAL STATE EXAMINATION

The Mini Mental State Examination (MMSE) is a test of cognition. It was first introduced by Folstein and colleagues in 1975,[1] and has subsequently been widely used throughout the world. This test is useful for distinguishing patients with organic and functional psychiatric illness. For example, a depressive illness can present a picture called pseudo-dementia, and because the MMSE is a useful measure of cognitive function it could differentiate this from depression.

### Scoring

The MMSE is administered by an interviewer. It has two parts – verbal and performance – and it covers the following domains:

▶ orientation to time and place, 10 points
▶ registration, 3 points
▶ attention and calculation, 5 points
▶ word recall, 3 points
▶ language, 8 points
▶ visual construction, 1 point.

The total possible score ranges from 0 to 30. A score of 24–30 indicates that there is no cognitive impairment, a score of 18–23 indicates mild to moderate cognitive impairment, and a score of < 17 indicates severe cognitive impairment. Although a low score suggests cognitive impairment, it is not diagnostic of the dementia syndrome or its subtypes.

The MMSE can be administered in survey settings by non-professionals. It is quick and practical to use.

### Administration time

It takes 5 to 10 minutes to administer this test.

### Reliability and validity

The MMSE has high criterion-related validity and reliability.[1] It correlates well with clinical diagnostic criteria such as DSM-III diagnosis and also radiological investigations (it correlates with cerebral atrophy on CT of the brain).[2] The MMSE is also sensitive to changes in condition over time. It has satisfactory inter-rater and test–retest reliability,[2] so is superior to the AMT. The MMSE is sufficiently validated when age, education and socio-economic status are taken into account.[2] Its sensitivity is lower in community samples than in clinic or hospital samples, because the prevalence of dementia in the former setting is lower. At a cut-off value of 23–24, its sensitivity is 30–60% and its specificity is 92–100%.[3] The low sensitivity suggests that this test is not effective in detecting mild or early dementia.

### Clinical applications

The strengths of the MMSE are its simplicity and ease of use by non-professionals. The instructions for scoring are short and standardised. The test has become the 'gold standard' screening instrument for detecting cognitive impairment in elderly people, and is now available in a number of languages, including Hindi, Gujarati, Punjabi, Urdu, Chinese, Bengali and African-Caribbean. Various population norms have been reproduced.[4] UK community prevalence estimates of cognitive impairment measured using the MMSE range from 3.9–5.4% for moderate to severe impairment to 8.5–9.8% for mild impairment, with higher rates in very old populations.[5] The MMSE is also used as a quantitative measure of cognitive impairment to monitor a change, and has been used as an assessment tool for monitoring patients who have been prescribed anti-dementia drugs. The test has been used in both hospital and community settings.

### Limitations

The results can be influenced by the respondent's socio-demographic background, including their ethnic origin and level of education. Thus people in lower social classes and with lower levels of education, even when not showing cognitive decline, are more likely to have lower scores,[6] whereas intelligent patients may have cognitive impairment even though they score 24 or above.[7] Cognitive dysfunction in some areas may be obscure. Patients with language impairment, visual and sensory impairment, or poor command of the English language may have low scores. It should be kept in mind that cognitive function, including MMSE score, declines with age. The rate of decline for individuals over 75 years is of the order of 1.3 points per year. One major limitation of the MMSE is that it tests very specific areas of cognition, including orientation, recall and praxis. The areas that are not assessed include long-term memory, and non-verbal and executive functions, such as goal selection, planning, motor sequencing and selective attention. The MMSE could miss mild cases of dementia. The test may be too global to detect clinically important changes, and ceiling effects and high false negative rates may be a problem.

Despite its limitations, the MMSE is the leading screening instrument for cognitive impairment. It has been recommended as one of the first-stage assessment scales for case finding in elderly people by the Royal College of Physicians and the British Geriatrics Society.[8]

### Modified versions

Alternative words can be chosen for the registration/recall items ('apple', 'table' and 'penny' are normally used, but alternatives include 'ball', 'flag', 'tree', 'lemon', 'key' and 'balloon'). For attention and calculation, serial sevens are generally used, or alternatively the subject is asked to spell the word 'world' backwards. Several modifications have been suggested for the MMSE, and a standardised version (the SMMSE) has been proposed,[9] especially for use in multi-centre research studies. The SMMSE contains more specific instructions, requires the subject to spell the word 'world' backwards, and has less inter- and intra-rater variance.

In summary, the MMSE is still the most widely used test for cognitive assessment of older adults, and remains the standard against which other mental status tests are measured. It is universally well known to clinicians.

## MMSE scale: guidelines for use

- Ensure that glasses or hearing aids are worn if appropriate.
- Check whether the person has language problems or is hemiplegic, etc.
- Questions 1 to 5 test orientation to time. Answers to questions about the day, date, month and year can only be accepted as correct if they are accurate. Allow leeway for the change in seasons (e.g. March can be winter or spring, June can be spring or summer, September can be summer or autumn, December can be autumn or winter).
- Questions 6 to 10 test orientation to place. Answers must be precise, but further clarification may be needed.
- Questions 11 to 13 relate to memory registration. If the person has difficulty answering them, these questions should be repeated up to five times.
- Questions 14 to 18 test attention/concentration. One point is scored each time for a difference of 7, even if the previous answer was incorrect.
- Questions 19 to 21 test memory recall. There should be no prompting.
- Questions 22 to 24 test language expression. There should be no prompting. 'No ifs and buts – should be read only once.'
- Questions 25 to 27 test comprehension of complex commands. Emphasise the importance of listening to the whole command before doing anything. It should be a three-stage command.
- Question 29: spelling and grammar are not important.
- Question 30: diagram must show two intersecting pentagons each with five equal sides and five clear angles, and the intersection of two angles should form a diamond shape.
- Questions 1 to 5 and 19 to 21 are not confounded by intelligence, and should be particularly scrutinised.

▶ If some items on the test cannot be administered due to dysphasia, hemiplegia, etc. then 23 cannot be considered as the cut-off point.

▶ A score of < 10 may suggest moderate to severe cognitive impairment, but other symptoms must be present to confirm that the patient has a dementing illness.

---

**MINI MENTAL STATE EXAMINATION**

1. What day of the week is it?
2. What is the date today?
3. What is the month?
4. What is the season?
5. What is the year?
6. Where are we now?
7. What floor are we on? (upstairs or downstairs)
8. In which town are we?
9. In which county/district are we?
10. In which country are we?
11, 12, 13. I am going to name three objects. After I have finished, I want you to repeat them. Remember what they are, because I am going to ask you again later. Apple. Table. Penny.
14. Take away 7 from 100.
15. Take 7 away from the number you get.
16. Keep going until I tell you to stop.
17. What are the three words I asked you to repeat a while ago?
18. What is this? (pencil)
19. What is this? (watch)
20. Can you repeat 'No ifs, ands or buts'?
21. Take this piece of paper, fold it in half and put it on the floor.
22. Please do this (close your eyes).
23. Write a sentence of your choice on this piece of paper.
24. Copy this drawing.

Reproduced with the permission of Oxford University Press from Hope R, Longmore J, editors. *Oxford Handbook of Clinical Medicine*. 4th ed. Oxford: Oxford University Press; 1998.

## REFERENCES

1 Folstein MF, Folstein SE, McHugh PR. 'Mini-mental state': a practical method for grading the cognitive state of patients for the clinician. *J Psychiatr Res.* 1975; **12**: 189–98.

2 Tombaugh TN, McIntyre NJ. The Mini-Mental State Examination: a comprehensive review. *J Am Geriatr Soc.* 1992; **40**: 922–35.

3 Wind AW, Schellevis FG, Van Staveren G *et al.* Limitations of the Mini-Mental State Examination in diagnosing dementia in general practice. *Int J Geriatr Psychiatry.* 1997; **12**: 101–8.

4 Crum RM, Anthony JC, Bassett SS *et al.* Population-based norms for the Mini-Mental State Examination by age and educational level. *JAMA.* 1993; **269**: 2386–91.

5 Brayne C, Calloway P. The case identification of dementia in the community: a comparison of methods. *Int J Geriatr Psychiatry.* 1990; **5**: 309–16.

6 Anthony JC, Le Resche L, Niaz U *et al.* Limits of the 'Mini-Mental State' as a screening test for dementia and delirium among hospital patients. *Psychol Med.* 1982; **12**: 397–408.

7 Jaggor C, Clarke M, Andersen J *et al.* Misclassification of dementia by the Mini-Mental State Examination: are education and social class the only factors? *Age Ageing.* 1992; **21**: 404–11.

8 Royal College of Physicians of London and the British Geriatrics Society. *Standardised Assessment Scales for Elderly People. Report of joint workshops of the Research Unit of Royal College of Physicians of London and the British Geriatrics Society.* London: Royal College of Physicians of London; 1992.

9 Molloy DW, Alemayehu E, Roberts R. Reliability of a standardized Mini-Mental State Examination compared with the traditional Mini-Mental State Examination. *Am J Psychiatry.* 1991; **148**: 102–5.

## CLOCK DRAWING TEST

This test has been used as a screening test for cognitive impairment and dementia.[1] It is a useful adjunct to the AMT or MMSE. The Clock Drawing Test can also be used to assess the severity of dementia, and has been used to follow the response to cholinesterase inhibitors in dementia patients.[2] This test can assess a wide range of functions in addition to memory, including comprehension, planning, motor programming and executive control, global attention, visual memory and reconstruction, concentration and visuo-spatial representation. It can therefore be used as a measure of spatial dysfunction and neglect. The test reflects frontal and temporo-parietal functioning.

### Scoring

The standard method is to use a pre-drawn circle of diameter approximately 4 inches or 10 cm. The person is asked to draw a clock face, marking the hours and then the hands for a particular time. The instructions are as follows: 'This circle represents a clock face. Please put in numbers so that it looks like a clock, and then set the time to 10 minutes past 11.' The 11.10 test is useful as it includes both visual fields. The test is easy to use, and there is no time limit. It requires verbal understanding, memory, spatial knowledge and constructive skills. The drawing is interpreted by the clinician, and there is wide variation in the way in which results can be interpreted. Various scoring and interpretation methods have been suggested. The scoring system ranges from a simple nominal scale (right/wrong) to a 4-point scale,[3] 6-point scale,[4] 10-point scale,[5] or even detailed 22- and 31-point scoring. A 6-point scale[4] is scored as follows:

- no real attempt, 0 points
- approximately circular face, 1 point
- symmetry of number placement, 2 points
- correctness of numbers, 3 points
- presence of two hands, 4 points
- correct time setting, 5 points.

### Administration time

It takes about 2 minutes to administer the test.

### Reliability and validity

Clock drawing with a score range of 1–5 is strongly correlated with the MMSE. A score range of 1–31 in clock drawing can correctly classify 86% of patients with Alzheimer's disease and 92% of controls.[6] In a literature review of studies

Score

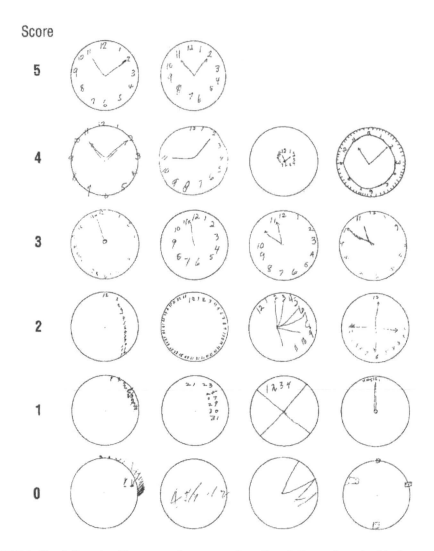

**FIGURE 1** Clock Drawing Test: severity scores from 5 to 0. Reproduced with the permission of John Wiley & Sons Ltd from Shulman KI. Clock drawing: is it the ideal cognitive screening test? *Int J Geriatr Psychiatry.* 2000; **15**: 548–61.

conducted between 1983 and 1998 using this test, the mean sensitivity and specificity were found to be 85%.[7] The test has high inter-rater and test–retest reliability and positive predictive value. It has good predictive validity and it complements the MMSE.[7]

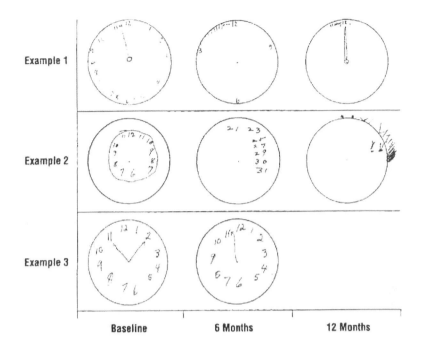

**FIGURE 2** Clock Drawing Test: sensitivity to deterioration in dementia. Reproduced with the permission of John Wiley & Sons Ltd from Shulman KI. Clock drawing: is it the ideal cognitive screening test? *Int J Geriatr Psychiatry.* 2000; **15**: 548–61.

### Clinical applications

A normal clock drawing reasonably excludes dementia. It is easy to document graphically in the patient's clinical records, and to record the changes over time in dementia patients. Respondents find the test interesting. It gives a good representation of distorted time, memory and perception. It is applicable across most cultures and language groups.

### Limitations

This test is unsuitable for people with visual impairments. In addition, the results can be influenced by level of education, age and the patient's mood. The value of the Clock Drawing Test in very early Alzheimer's disease is questionable. On its own it is unlikely to suffice as a screen for dementia.

In summary, overall the Clock Drawing Test is an important adjunct to the cognitive screening process and is sensitive to cognitive change.

## REFERENCES

1 Shulman K, Shedletsky R, Silver I. The challenge of time: clock drawing and cognitive function in the elderly. *Int J Geriatr Psychiatry.* 1986; 1: 135–40.

2 Brodaty H, Moore CM. The Clock Drawing Test for dementia of the Alzheimer's type: a comparison of three scoring methods in a memory disorders clinic. *Int J Geriatr Psychiatry.* 1997; 12: 619–27.

3 Death J, Douglas A, Kenny RA. Comparison of clock drawing with Mini Mental State Examination as a screening test in elderly acute hospital admissions. *Postgrad Med J.* 1993; 69: 696–700.

4 Shua-Haim J, Koppuzha G, Gross J et al. A simple scoring system for clock drawing in patients with Alzheimer's disease. *J Am Geriatr Soc.* 1996; 44: 335.

5 Manos PJ, Wu R. The ten-point clock test: a quick screen and grading method for cognitive impairment in medical and surgical patients. *Int J Psychiatry Med.* 1994; 24: 229–44.

6 Borson S, Brush M, Gil E et al. The Clock Drawing Test: utility for dementia detection in multi-ethnic elders. *J Gerontol.* 1999; 54: M534–40.

7 Shulman KI. Clock drawing: is it the ideal cognitive screening test? *Int J Geriatr Psychiatry.* 2000; 15: 548–61.

## CLIFTON ASSESSMENT PROCEDURE FOR THE ELDERLY

The Clifton Assessment Procedure for the Elderly (CAPE)[1] is widely used in geriatric and psychogeriatric settings. It developed as a result of research conducted at the Psychiatric Department, Clifton Hospital, York, in the UK. Initially designed for hospital populations, this scale has also been found to be useful for community services. It measures cognition as well as the behavioural competence of an individual, and is applicable in both clinical and research settings. It has been useful for assessment not only by psychologists but also by many other professionals who are involved in care for the elderly, such as social workers, health visitors, general practitioners, occupational therapists and clinicians.

### *Scoring*

The CAPE consists of two interrelated scales, each of which can be used alone or in combination:

▶ The Cognitive Assessment Scale (formerly known as the Clifton Assessment Scale) is a short psychological test. Little training is required to administer it, the test is brief, and it evaluates the existence and degree of impairment in mental functioning, rather than testing intelligence. This scale consists of three brief mental tests:[2]
  - the Information–Orientation Test, which has 12 questions designed to assess information and orientation
  - the Mental Abilities Test, which has 4 items that relate to skills of counting, saying the alphabet, writing one's name and reading. This reflects retention of the above four skills, levels of attention and concentration, evidence of visual defect and intellectual level
  - the Psychomotor Performance Test is the Gibson Spiral Maze with amended administration and scoring criteria. It involves the subject tracing a circular route with a pencil. It measures fine motor performance and hand–eye co-ordination. It identifies slowing of psychomotor performance over and above the deterioration associated with normal ageing.

▶ The Behaviour Rating Scale (BRS).[3] This is a shorter version of the Stockton Geriatric Rating Scale. It assesses physical dependency, communication and behaviour, and it can be filled in by an observer (e.g. a relative or member of staff) who is familiar with the subject's behaviour. It is useful for measuring behavioural problems in elderly patients with dementia. The BRS contains 18 items, four of which relate to mobility, continence and activities of daily living (ADL). The remaining items relate to confused behaviour. The scale asks about level of current functioning and about behaviour during the last 2 weeks. The range of possible scores is from 0 to 36, and a score of 18–36 indicates maximum dependency.

The cognitive scale is completed with the subject, and the behaviour scale is completed by a relative or care staff member. Information from both scales is recorded on separate summary sheets, known as the CAPE Report Form. The individual scores are evaluated against a 5-point grading system reflecting varying degrees of impairment. These represent varying degrees of care and support.

### Administration time
It takes 15–25 minutes to administer both scales.

### Reliability and validity
In large samples the CAPE has shown good reliability, high sensitivity and high specificity among psychiatric patients. It has mainly been tested in hospitalised patients.[4] Extensive inter-rater and test–retest reliability studies have been reported.[5] Validity has been tested against psychiatric diagnosis and hospital discharge and also with other mental status tests.[6]

### Clinical applications
These include the following:
- Clinical assessment:
  - diagnosis – the CAPE can separate functional psychiatric disorders from organic brain disease. It can be used to identify dementia
  - prognosis – the CAPE identifies future management needs and prognosis. CAPE scores predict the likelihood of hospital discharge.
- Need for placement – the BRS is useful in hospital, allowing identification of dependency and placement needs. It can also reduce inappropriate admission delays and inappropriate placement.
- Identification of patients for rehabilitation.
- Evaluation of effects of therapeutic intervention.

The CAPE can be applied in hospital, home or nursing home settings. It is generally administered by nurses, especially psychiatric nurses. The advantage of this instrument is that it provides a common metric across different settings based on a person's degree of impairment and dependency. It can be used in various combinations, ranging from full assessment battery to a brief CAPE survey. Each of these scales provides information about the level of care related to disease and disability in older age. Thus the CAPE provides practical information that is useful when planning service provision. Because it is easy to administer, the CAPE is widely used in the UK.

*Note:* The author could not obtain permission to reproduce the CAPE scale in this book. For a copy of the complete scale, the reader is referred to *The Manual of the Clifton Assessment Procedures for the Elderly (CAPE)*.[1] To obtain permission to reproduce the scale, the reader should contact Hodder and Stoughton Educational, 338 Euston Road, London NW13BH.

## REFERENCES

1 Pattie AH, Gilleard CJ. *Manual of the Clifton Assessment Procedures for the Elderly (CAPE).* Sevenoaks: Hodder and Stoughton Educational; 1979.

2 Gibson HB. *Manual to the Gibson Spiral Maze.* 2nd ed. Sevenoaks: Hodder and Stoughton Educational; 1978.

3 Gilleard CJ, Pattie AH. The Stockton Geriatric Rating Scale: a shortened version with British normative data. *Br J Psychiatry.* 1977; **131**: 90–4.

4 McPherson FM, Gamsu CV, Kiemle G *et al.* The concurrent validity of the survey version of the Clifton Assessment Procedure for the Elderly. *Br J Clin Psychol.* 1985; **24**: 83–91.

5 Mulgrave NW. CAPE. In: Keyser DJ, Sweetland RC, editors. *Test Critiques. Volume II.* Kansas City, MO: Test Corporation of America; 1985.

6 Pattie A, Gilleard C. A brief psychogeriatric assessment schedule. Validation against psychiatric diagnosis and discharge from hospital. *Br J Psychiatry.* 1975; **127**: 489–93.

## BARTHEL INDEX

The Barthel Index (BI) was first introduced by Mahoney and Barthel in 1965,[1] and is now extensively used in rehabilitation. It was initially developed to measure functional ability before and after treatment and to assess the amount of nursing care needed. Initially it was designed for use with long-stay hospitalised patients with neuromuscular or musculoskeletal problems.[1] It has subsequently been used and applied to evaluate treatment outcomes. It is extremely popular, and is one of the oldest and most widely used tests.

### *Scoring*

The BI is based on a rating scale that is completed by an observer. It covers personal toileting, feeding, mobility from bed to chair, transfers, bathing, walking, dressing, incontinence and going upstairs. A total of 10 activities are scored, and the values are then added to give a total score ranging from 0 (totally dependent) to 100 (completely independent). Lower scores indicate greater dependency.

According to Sinoff and Ore,[2] scoring on the BI can be interpreted as follows:

▶ score of 80–100, independent
▶ score of 60–79, needs minimal help with ADL
▶ score of 40–59, partially dependent
▶ score of 20–39, very dependent
▶ score of < 20, totally dependent.

The BI measures what the patient *actually* does rather than what they *can* do. Information is obtained via verbal reports from patients, carers and staff, and by direct observation of some activities.

### *Administration time*

It takes about 10 minutes to administer the test.

### *Reliability and validity*

The BI is sensitive, has concurrent and predictive validity, and is reliable.[1] It has good inter-rater, test–retest, and reported or observed reliability.[3] The internal consistency of the BI is extremely high, with a Cronbach's alpha coefficient of 0.98.[4] Intra-observer and inter-observer reliabilities are high, with a Pearson's r score ranging from 0.89 to 0.99.[4] Telephone assessments of the BI using structured interviews have shown high correlations with direct measurements.[4] However, purely self-reported scores tend to be less accurate than direct measurements, especially in patients with cognitive dysfunction or serious illness, and in those over 75 years of age.[2] The BI has proven value in discriminating between groups of patients (construct validity) and predicting outcome (predictive validity).[5] Around 70% of patients with a score of < 40 had died or were living in long-term facilities, and 94% of patients with a score of 80–100 were living in the community 6 months post stroke.[5] Moreover, patients with stroke who had a score of > 60 after rehabilitation were more likely to be active in their homes and communities, to have more social interaction and to be more satisfied with life than those with scores of ≤ 60.[5] The scale correlates with clinical impression (e.g. motor loss following stroke). It also correlates well with various prognostic scores of stroke patients, and with other scales (e.g. PULSES Profile score and Edinburgh Rehabilitation Status Scale score).[6]

### Clinical applications

The BI measures activities of daily living (ADL). It taps more functional items than other scales in that it includes items such as ability to walk up stairs. It is simple to use and easily communicated. The BI is useful for repeatedly assessing improvements in patients over time in order to determine the effectiveness of rehabilitation therapies.[5] The scale is suitable for hospital patients as well as those living at home. In clinical geriatric practice the assessment of premorbid BI is useful for setting goals, monitoring progress and making discharge plans. It also covers continence, unlike the Rivermead ADL Scale. A low score indicates a low likelihood of discharge home, poor outcome after stroke and a lower level of social and domestic activities. Many investigators are familiar with the BI, which is advantageous in multi-centre studies. Its high reliability even with telephone assessments makes this tool especially useful when studying patients who are unable to return for face-to-face follow-up assessments.

### Limitations

The scale has been criticised with regard to its usefulness in community settings. If it is used in the community, it needs to include everyday life tasks such as cooking, shopping, and so on. Many aspects of functional independence are not included, such as cognition, language, visual function, emotional impairment and pain. Each of these components could have a significant effect on a person's independence. Moreover, scoring may be location dependent. Some domestic tasks, role functioning, socio-psychological functioning, mental status and general well-being are not represented. The scale is also insensitive to small differences. Furthermore, self-reports could differ from therapist ratings.

The scale suffers from 'ceiling effects' – that is, the maximum score can be achieved by a disabled person, and therefore it does not differentiate disability well among patients with higher levels of functioning. For example, although a score of 100 means independence in all 10 areas, a person with this score may not be able to live alone, and assistance in instrumental activities of daily living (IADL) (e.g. cooking, housework) may still be required. A stroke patient with aphasia may be completely normal with regard to all items of the BI, yet be unable to function outside the home without the assistance of another person. The BI also has 'floor effects' and is not useful in the setting of acute stroke. This is because most patients even with minor stroke are bed bound for the first few hours after stroke, either due to deficit or because of a medical directive, and will therefore have low scores. For this reason the BI cannot be used to measure initial stroke severity.

Use of the summary score from the BI is not always appropriate. As the BI reflects function in two areas (i.e. self-care and mobility) together, use of the summary score blurs the distinction between these two areas. Furthermore, the BI is neither a metric nor a true ordinal scale, and scores should not be interpreted as percentages. For example, an individual who scores 50 should not be assumed to be functioning at 50% of the level of independence of an individual who has a score of 100.

## MODIFIED 20-POINT BARTHEL INDEX

This scale was introduced by Collin and colleagues in 1988,[7] and is also a measure of ADL.

### *Scoring*

This scale gives a maximum score of 20. The scoring is simple, with scores ranging from 0 to 2 or 3 for each activity. Depending on the score, the patient can be placed within arbitrary broad categories of disability (e.g. a score of < 4 indicates total dependence and a score of < 12 indicates dependence). However, rather than using these 'thresholds', outcome measurements are better described using 'grouping scores' – that is, comparisons made between patients with an initial very low score (< 4), low score (5–8), interim score (9–11) and high score (≥ 12). In general the assessment is made by the nurse or clinician describing what the patient *actually* does rather than what they *can* do. It also reflects the amount of assistance that the patient needs.

### *Administration time*

It takes about 30 seconds to administer the test.

### *Validity and reliability*

The modified 20–point BI is valid and reliable even in stroke patients.[8] Changes in the scale correlate well with physician assessment of progress.

### *Clinical applications*

The modified 20–point BI is easier and quicker to administer than the 100-point BI. Patients with higher scores should also preferably be assessed using a scale of IADL (e.g. the Nottingham Extended ADL or the Frenchay Activities Index). This provides information about the handicap experienced by the patient.

There is wide experience of the use of the 20-point BI in all hospital settings. It has been widely utilised in the elderly, even in frail patients and those suffering from a wide range of chronic conditions that cause disability. Scores on this scale have been shown to correlate with length of hospital stay, mortality, independence at home and place of discharge. In stroke patients there is a predictable progression through the items as recovery occurs.[8] The 20-point BI can reflect change in a patient at the beginning and end of an admission, but subtle changes during hospitalisation are not always reflected in the score.

### Limitations

The changes do not reflect equivalent changes in disability across different activities. The 20-point BI is not a continuous scale, as one point change at the top of the scale cannot be equated with one point change at the bottom of the scale (e.g. a change in score from 10 to 18 does not necessarily mean the same as a change from 2 to 10). Furthermore, the changes can occur beyond the scale points (the so-called 'floor' and 'ceiling' effects). A patient who achieves the maximum score on the scale may not necessarily be able to function fully and without handicap or disability. Moreover, a score of 0 covers a wide range. It is insensitive to small differences. The scale is limited to physical activities and does not take into account mental status or social well-being. It only measures one aspect of quality of life, and it omits domestic, social and other role functioning (work, parenting, etc.). As it measures what the patient *actually* does rather than what they *can* do, scoring may be location dependent. Respondents who walk independently with a frame or stick or without aids will score the same.

Despite its limitations, the 20-point BI is one of the briefest assessments of basic ADL currently available, and has become one of the most widely known ADL instruments, especially in the UK. It is recommended by the Royal College of Physicians for routine use in the assessment of older people.[9]

Other modifications to the 100-point BI include Granger's modified BI and Gompertz's modified BI.[10]

---

**MODIFIED 20-POINT BARTHEL INDEX**

Bowels
- Incontinent (or needs enema), 0 points
- Occasional accident (once a week), 1 point
- Continent, 2 points

Bladder
- Incontinent or catheterised, 0 points
- Occasional accident, 1 point
- Continent (for over 7 days), 2 points

Grooming
- Needs help, 0 points
- Independent, 1 point

Toilet use
- Dependent, 0 points

---

- Needs some help, 1 point
- Independent, 2 points

Feeding
- Unable to feed, 0 points
- Needs help, 1 point
- Independent, 2 points

Transfer
- Unable to transfer, 0 points
- Needs major help (1 to 2 people), 1 point
- Needs minor help, 2 points
- Independent, 3 points

Mobility
- Immobile, 0 points
- Wheel chair independent, 1 point
- Walks with help of 1 person, 2 points
- Independent (may use aid, e.g. walking stick), 3 points

Dressing
- Dependent, 0 points
- Needs help, 1 point
- Independent, 2 points

Stairs
- Unable to use stairs, 0 points
- Needs help, 1 point
- Independent, 2 points

Bathing
- Dependent, 0 points
- Independent (unsupervised), 1 point

Reproduced with the permission of Professor DT Wade.

## Guidelines for use of 20-point Barthel Index

▶ The Barthel Index should record what the patient *does*, not what they *could do*.

▶ Information is obtained from verbal report (from patient, carer or staff) together with direct observation of activities.

▶ The patient's performance is established using the best available evidence. Direct testing is not always necessary.

▶ The aim is to establish the *degree of independence* from any help, physical or verbal, however minor and for whatever reason.

▶ The need for supervision means that the patient is *not* independent.

▶ Usually performance during the preceding 24 to 48 hours is important (or during the preceding week for bowel and bladder).

▶ Unconscious patients should be given a score of 0.

▶ The use of aids for independence is allowed.

▶ Bowels: If the patient needs an enema from the nurse, they are deemed to be incontinent.

▶ Bladder: a catheterised patient who can manage their catheter alone is deemed to be 'continent.' An 'occasional' bladder accident is defined as < 1 per day.

▶ Grooming includes brushing teeth, doing hair, washing face, fitting false teeth and shaving. Implements can be provided by the helper.

▶ Toilet use: 'independent' means able to reach the toilet/commode, undress, clean oneself, dress and leave.

▶ Feeding: 'help' is defined as having food cut up and feeding oneself.

▶ Transfer: means from bed to chair and back. If the patient has no sitting balance they should be given a score of 0.

▶ Mobility: this refers to mobility indoors. The patient may use an aid.

▶ Dressing: clothes could be adapted. 'Help' is defined as assistance with dress/button/zip.

▶ Bathing: this is the most difficult activity. 'Independent' is defined as unsupervised and unaided.

### REFERENCES

1 Mahoney FI, Barthel DW. Functional evaluation: the Barthel Index. *Md State Med J.* 1965; 14: 61–5.

2 Sinoff G, Ore L. The Barthel Activities of Daily Living Index: self-reporting versus actual performance in the old-old (> 75 years). *J Am Geriatr Soc.* 1997; 45: 832–6.

3 Fricke J, Unsworth CA. Inter-rater reliability of the original and modified Barthel Index, and a comparison with the Functional Independence Measure. *Austr Occup Ther J.* 1997; 44: 22–9.

4 Shinar D, Gross CR, Bronstein KS *et al.* Reliability of the activities of daily living scale and its use in telephone interview. *Arch Phys Med Rehabil.* 1987; **68**: 723–8.

5 Granger CV, Dewis LS, Petrs NC *et al.* Stroke rehabilitation: analysis of repeated Barthel Index measures. *Arch Phys Med Rehabil.* 1979; **60**: 14–17.

6 Granger CV, Albrecht GL, Hamilton BB. Outcome of comprehensive medical rehabilitation: measurement by PULSES Profile and the Barthel Index. *Arch Phys Med Rehabil.* 1979; **60**: 145–54.

7 Collin C, Wade DT, Davies S *et al.* The Barthel ADL Index: a reliability study. *Int Disabil Stud.* 1988; **10**: 61–3.

8 Kalra L, Crome P. The role of prognostic scores in targeting stroke rehabilitation in elderly patients. *J Am Geriatr Soc.* 1993; **41**: 396–400.

9 Royal College of Physicians of London and the British Geriatrics Society. *Standardised Assessment Scales for Elderly People. Report of joint workshops of the Research Unit of Royal College of Physicians of London and the British Geriatrics Society.* London: Royal College of Physicians of London; 1992.

10 Gompertz P, Pound P, Ebrahim S. The reliability of stroke outcome measures. *Clin Rehabil.* 1993; **7**: 290–96.

## NOTTINGHAM EXTENDED ACTIVITIES OF
## DAILY LIVING QUESTIONNAIRE

This scale was introduced by Nouri and Lincoln in 1987,[1] and has 22 items arranged in four sections. It is an interviewer-administered questionnaire. Four-point responses are scored 0 or 1, where 0 indicates 'major difficulties' and 1 indicates 'on my own.' It covers mobility, kitchen tasks, other domestic tasks and leisure activities. The level of activity is assessed – that is, whether the subject *does* the activity rather than whether they *can* do it.[2] A modified Gompertz's Nottingham Questionnaire is also available.[3]

---

Name of patient: ...............................................................

Form filled in by patient?    Yes ☐  No ☐

If no, please state your name and relationship to the patient.

.........................................................................

Please tick one box only for each and every question on this page.

For these questions please record only WHAT YOU HAVE ACTUALLY DONE IN THE LAST WEEK OR SO (*not* what you think you could do, ought to do or would like to do).

| | | No | With help | On my own with difficulty | On my own |
|---|---|---|---|---|---|
| a. | Do you walk around outside? | ☐ | ☐ | ☐ | ☐ |
| b. | Do you climb stairs? | ☐ | ☐ | ☐ | ☐ |
| c. | Do you get in and out of the car? | ☐ | ☐ | ☐ | ☐ |
| d. | Do you walk over uneven ground? | ☐ | ☐ | ☐ | ☐ |
| e. | Do you cross roads? | ☐ | ☐ | ☐ | ☐ |
| f. | Do you travel on public transport? | ☐ | ☐ | ☐ | ☐ |
| g. | Do you manage to feed yourself? | ☐ | ☐ | ☐ | ☐ |

---

| | | No | With help | On my own with difficulty | On my own |
|---|---|---|---|---|---|
| h. | Do you manage to make yourself a hot drink? | ☐ | ☐ | ☐ | ☐ |
| i. | Do you take hot drinks from one room to another? | ☐ | ☐ | ☐ | ☐ |
| j. | Do you do the washing up? | ☐ | ☐ | ☐ | ☐ |
| k. | Do you make yourself a hot snack? | ☐ | ☐ | ☐ | ☐ |
| l. | Do you manage your own money when you are out? | ☐ | ☐ | ☐ | ☐ |
| m. | Do you wash small items of clothing? | ☐ | ☐ | ☐ | ☐ |
| n. | Do you do your own housework? | ☐ | ☐ | ☐ | ☐ |
| o. | Do you do your own shopping? | ☐ | ☐ | ☐ | ☐ |
| p. | Do you do a full clothes wash? | ☐ | ☐ | ☐ | ☐ |
| q. | Do you read newspapers or books? | ☐ | ☐ | ☐ | ☐ |
| r. | Do you use the telephone? | ☐ | ☐ | ☐ | ☐ |
| s. | Do you write letters? | ☐ | ☐ | ☐ | ☐ |
| t. | Do you go out socially? | ☐ | ☐ | ☐ | ☐ |
| u. | Do you manage your own garden? | ☐ | ☐ | ☐ | ☐ |
| v. | Do you drive a car? | ☐ | ☐ | ☐ | ☐ |

Reproduced with the permission of Professor Nadina Lincoln, Nottingham, from Nouri FM, Lincoln NB. An extended activities of daily living scale for stroke patients. *Clin Rehabil.* 1987; **1**: 301–5.

## REFERENCES

1 Nouri FM, Lincoln NB. An extended activities of daily living scale for stroke patients. *Clin Rehabil.* 1987; **1**: 301–5.

2 Lincoln NB, Gladman JRF. The extended activities of daily living scale: a further validation. *Disabil Rehabil.* 1992; **14**: 41–3.

3 Gompertz P, Pound P, Ebrahim S. *Kudo: a kit for describing the outcome of stroke.* London: Department of Public Health, Royal Free Hospital Medical School; 1993.

## RANKIN HANDICAP SCALE

This scale was developed in 1957 by Rankin for stroke patients, to assess the resulting disability.[1] Several versions of the scale are available. Rankin scales measure independence rather than being task oriented, giving a better impression of self-care than disability indexes such as the Barthel Index, and thus representing handicap rather than disability. The Rankin Handicap Scale is quick to use and is completed by health professionals. The scale has five grades (see box below).[1]

---

Grade I:  No significant disability: able to carry out all activities.

Grade II:  Slight disability: unable to carry out some of previous activities, but able to look after own affairs without assistance.

Grade III:  Moderate disability: requiring some help, but able to walk without assistance.

Grade IV:  Moderately severe disability: unable to walk without assistance, and unable to attend to own bodily needs without assistance.

Grade V:  Severe disability: bedridden, incontinent and requiring constant nursing care and attention.

Reproduced with the permission of the *Scottish Medical Journal* from Rankin J. Cerebral vascular accidents in patients over the age of 60. II. Prognosis. *Scott Med J.* 1957; **2**: 200–15.

---

## MODIFIED RANKIN SCALE

The modified Rankin Scale (mRS) was published by Van Swieten and colleagues in 1988.[2] It measures functional independence, incorporating the WHO components of body function, activity and participation. The mRS represents *handicap* rather than disability.

### Scoring

There are six grades in total (see box below), including Grade 0. The scale is completed by a healthcare professional. A one-point shift in this scale is clinically significant because of large category sizes, so recording should be as accurate as possible. Patients may use adaptive devices and still be considered independent, but the need for supervision or even minimum aid from another person is scored as dependent.

Grade 0: No symptoms.

Grade 1: No significant disability despite symptoms; able to carry out all usual duties and activities.

Grade 2: Slight disability; unable to carry out ALL previous activities, but able to look after own affairs without assistance.

Grade 3: Moderate disability; requiring some help, but able to walk without assistance.

Grade 4: Moderately severe disability; unable to walk without assistance, and unable to attend to own bodily needs without assistance.

Grade 5: Severe disability; bedridden, incontinent and requiring constant nursing care and attention.

Reproduced with the permission of Lippincott, Williams and Wilkins from Van Swieten JC, Koudstaal PJ, Visser MC *et al.* Inter-observer agreement for the assessment of handicap in stroke patients. *Stroke.* 1988; **19**: 604–7.

### Administration time

It takes around 30 seconds to administer this scale.

### Reliability and validity

The inter-rater reliability and validity of the mRS in stroke outcome has been well established.[3] This scale has moderate concurrent validity with infarct volumes, with correlation coefficients of 0.4–0.5,[4] which is similar to the Barthel Index and other functional disability scales. The construct validity of the mRS shows excellent agreement with other rating scales.[3] In a prospective study comparing several outcome measures in patients after ischaemic stroke, it was noted that the mRS was more responsive to changes in functional status, and a better instrument for differentiating between changes in mild to moderate disability, especially after mild stroke, than the Barthel Index, probably because there was less ceiling effect.[5] The mRS is also more reflective of disability in an emotional context, because it is more susceptible to change by depression.

### Clinical applications

Rankin scales have been used extensively in stroke research. They are based on the level of mobility, and thus measure impairments and disabilities. Both scales are simple to use. They are very useful in busy clinical settings, and allow rapid assessment of the effect of stroke on patients' activities and their participation in a social context. Data from the Glycine Antagonist in Neuroprotection (GAIN) International Trial[6] were used to explore the patterns and extent of treatment effect and to estimate statistical power for a range of end points with the mRS or Barthel Index. The mRS end points needed substantially smaller sample sizes to achieve adequate statistical power, and the odds of achieving a statistically significant result increased by 89% with the mRS end point compared with the BI end point.[6] Analysis across the distribution of scores rather than dichotomisation maximises the usefulness of the mRS.[7] The simplicity of the mRS can affect its reliability, as rating scales with more items or rankings can offer higher reliability.[3] A structured interview has been proposed to improve its inter-rater reliability.[8] It was shown that with a structured interview the unweighted k value was 0.74 with agreement in 81% of cases, compared with a value of 0.25 without structured interview.[8] Additional methods to improve the reliability of the mRS continue to be developed.[9]

### Limitations

The mRS has low sensitivity. The overall responsiveness of this scale is poor over short-term intervals (e.g. from admission to discharge) at least in part because a substantial clinical threshold exists between each point in the scale, and because patients have not resumed their usual roles and activities while in hospital.[5] Moreover, the mRS is a broad-based measure and lacks specificity. Certain domains, such as cognition, language, visual function, emotional impairment and pain, are not directly measured. A small stroke or mild neurological disability (e.g. a visual field defect causing a truck driver to become unemployed, or post-stroke depression hampering normal activities) can lead to severe disability. Furthermore, a large stroke can result in mild disability (e.g. cerebellar stroke in a sedentary person). In acute stroke, the mRS can have a floor effect (e.g. patients can have high scores, suggesting severe disability, because most patients are bedbound for the first few hours after stroke).[5] There is no substitute for assessing full-scale functional ability, such as that used in research studies.

## Structured interview for the Modified Rankin Scale

The purpose of the structured interview is to assign mRS grades to patients in a systematic way.[8] The interview consists of five sections corresponding to the levels of disability on the mRS. Use of the structured interview improves agreement between raters in their assessment of the mRS after stroke.[8]

### *Interview*

▶ Use the best source of information available (either the patient him- or herself or a person who is familiar with the patient).
▶ Please mark (X) in the appropriate box.
▶ Record responses to all questions.
▶ If the problem/limitation existed before the stroke, mark 'Yes' in the 'Before stroke' column and proceed to the next item.

| STRUCTURED INTERVIEW FOR THE MODIFIED RANKIN SCALE | | | |
|---|---|---|---|
| **1** | **Constant care** | | |
| | | *Now* | *Before stroke* |
| 1.1 | Does the person require constant care? | Yes (5) No | Yes No |
| **2** | **Assistance with attending to bodily needs/walking** | | |
| | | *Now* | *Before stroke* |
| 2.1 | Is assistance essential for eating? | Yes (4) No | Yes No |
| 2.2 | Is assistance essential for using the toilet? | Yes (4) No | Yes No |
| 2.3 | Is assistance essential for routine hygiene? | Yes (4) No | Yes No |
| 2.4 | Is assistance essential for walking? | Yes (4) No | Yes No |
| **3** | **Assistance with looking after own affairs** | | |
| | | *Now* | *Before stroke* |
| 3.1 | Is assistance essential for preparing a simple meal? | Yes (3) No | Yes No |

| | | | |
|------|-----------------------------------------------------------------|-------------|--------|
| 3.2 | Is assistance essential for basic household chores? | Yes (3) No | Yes No |
| 3.3 | Is assistance essential for looking after household expenses? | Yes (3) No | Yes No |
| 3.4 | Is assistance essential for local travel? | Yes (3) No | Yes No |
| 3.5 | Is assistance essential for local shopping? | Yes (3) No | Yes No |

| | | | |
|--------|-----------------------------------------------------------------------------------------------------------------------|-----|-----|
| **4** | **Usual duties and activities** | | |
| **4.1** | **Work** | | |
| 4.1.1 | Before stroke, was the person working or seeking work (or studying as a student)? | Yes | No |
| 4.1.2 | Since stroke, has there been a change in the person's ability to do work or study? | Yes | No |
| | If 'yes', how restricted are they? | | |
| | Reduced levels of work (e.g. change from full-time to part-time or change in level of responsibility). (2) | | |
| | Currently unable to work. (2) | | |
| **4.2** | **Family responsibilities** | | |
| 4.2.1 | Before stroke, was the person looking after family at home? | Yes | No |
| 4.2.2 | Since stroke, has there been a change in their ability to look after family at home? | Yes | No |
| | If 'yes', how restricted are they? | | |
| | Reduced responsibility for looking after family. (2) | | |
| | Currently unable to look after family. (2) | | |
| **4.3** | **Social and leisure activities** | Yes | No |
| 4.3.1 | Before stroke, did the person have regular free-time activities? | Yes | No |
| 4.3.2 | Since stroke, has there been a change in their ability to participate in these activities? | Yes | No |
| | If 'yes', how restricted are they? | | |
| | Participate a bit less: at least half as often as before the stroke. | | |

| | | | |
|---|---|---|---|
| 4.3.2 | Participate much less: less than half as often. (2) | Yes | No |
| | Unable to take participate: rarely, if ever, take part. (2) | | |
| **4.4** | **Family and friendships** | Yes | No |
| 4.4.1 | Since the stroke, has the person had problems with relationships or become isolated? | Yes | No |
| | If 'yes', what is the extent of disruption/ strain? | | |
| | Occasional – less than weekly | | |
| | Frequent – once a week or more, but tolerable. (2) | | |
| | Constant – daily and intolerable. (2) | | |
| 4.4.2 | Before stroke, were any similar problems present? | Yes | No |

| | | | |
|---|---|---|---|
| **5** | **Symptoms as a result of the stroke** | | |
| 5.1 | Does the patient have any symptoms resulting from stroke? | Yes (1) | No |

| | | Now | Before stroke |
|---|---|---|---|
| 5.2 | *Symptom checklist* | *Now* | *Before stroke* |
| 5.2.1 | Does the person have difficulty reading or writing? | Yes (1) No | Yes No |
| 5.2.2 | Does the person have difficulty speaking or finding the right word? | Yes (1) No | Yes No |
| 5.2.3 | Does the person have problems with balance or coordination? | Yes (1) No | Yes No |
| 5.2.4 | Does the person have visual problems? | Yes (1) No | Yes No |
| 5.2.5 | Does the person have numbness (in face, arms, legs, hands or feet)? | Yes (1) No | Yes No |
| 5.2.6 | Has the person experienced loss of movement (in face, arms, legs, hands or feet)? | Yes (1) No | Yes No |
| 5.2.7 | Does the person have difficulty with swallowing? | Yes (1) No | Yes No |

| 5.2.8 | Are there any other symptoms? (Please record: ..................... ................................. | Yes (1) No | Yes No |

Reproduced with the permission of Professor Lindsay Wilson from: Wilson L *et al. Stroke.* 2005; **36**: 777–81.

## REFERENCES

1 Rankin J. Cerebral vascular accidents in patients over the age of 60. II. Prognosis. *Scott Med J.* 1957; **2**: 200–15.

2 Van Swieten JC, Koudstaal PJ, Visser MC *et al.* Inter-observer agreement for the assessment of handicap in stroke patients. *Stroke.* 1988; **19**: 604–7.

3 Streiner DL, Norman GR. *Health Measurement Scales. A practical guide to their development and use.* 2nd ed. Oxford: Oxford University Press; 1995. pp. 111–12.

4 Schiemanck SK, Post MWM, Kwakkel G *et al.* Ischaemic lesion volume correlates with long-term functional outcome and quality of life of middle cerebral artery stroke survivors. *Restor Neurol Neurosci.* 2005; **23**: 257–63.

5 Dromerick AW, Edwards DF, Diringer MN. Sensitivity to changes in disability after stroke: a comparison of four scales useful in clinical trials. *J Rehabil Res Dev.* 2003; **40**: 1–8.

6 Young FB, Lees KR, Weir CJ for the Glycine Antagonist in Neuroprotection (GAIN) International Trial Steering Committee and Investigators. Strengthening acute stroke trials through optimal use of disability end points. *Stroke.* 2003; **34**: 2676–80.

7 Lai S-M, Duncan PW. Stroke recovery profile and the modified Rankin assessment. *Neuroepidemiology.* 2001; **20**: 26–30.

8 Wilson JTL, Hareendran A, Hendry A *et al.* Reliability of the modified Rankin Scale across multiple raters: benefits of a structured interview. *Stroke.* 2005; **36**: 777–81.

9 Shinohara Y, Minematsu K, Amano T *et al.* Modified Rankin Scale with expanded guidance scheme and interview questionnaire: inter-rater agreement and reproducibility of assessment. *Cerebrovasc Dis.* 2006; **21**: 271–8.

## FUNCTIONAL INDEPENDENCE MEASURE AND FUNCTIONAL ASSESSMENT MEASURE

### Functional Independence Measure

The Functional Independence Measure (FIM) scale assesses physical and cognitive disability.[1] This scale focuses on the burden of care – that is, the level of disability indicating the burden of caring for them.

### Scoring

Items are scored on the level of assistance required for an individual to perform activities of daily living. The scale includes 18 items, of which 13 items are physical domains based on the Barthel Index and 5 items are cognition items. Each item is scored from 1 to 7 based on level of independence, where 1 represents total dependence and 7 indicates complete independence. The scale can be administered by a physician, nurse, therapist or layperson. Possible scores range from 18 to 126, with higher scores indicating more independence. Alternatively, 13 physical items could be scored separately from 5 cognitive items.

### Time

It takes 1 hour to train a rater to use the FIM scale, and 30 minutes to score the scale for each patient.

### Clinical application

The FIM scale is used to measure the patient's progress and assess rehabilitation outcomes. This scale is useful in clinical settings of rehabilitation. The FIM was carefully designed and developed with the consensus of the US National Advisory Committee, with close attention to definitions, administration and reliability. Manuals, training and videos are provided (further information can be found at www.udsmr.org). The FIM has been used in a number of countries, including the USA, Canada, Australia, France, Japan, Sweden and Germany. Studies of large samples have been published, including a study of 93 829 subjects.[2] The FIM has been used extensively in rehabilitation, including that for stroke and multiple sclerosis. Scores are responsive to change and also reflect the patient's discharge destination.

### FIM and FAM

The Functional Assessment Measure (FAM) includes FIM items but also adds 12 new items, mainly covering cognition, such as community integration, emotional status, orientation, attention, reading and writing skills, and employability.[3] The FIM scale on its own had ceiling effects, so the FAM was proposed, which extends the coverage of the FIM. This scale was originally intended for patients with brain injury, but is in fact useful in all rehabilitation settings.

FIM + FAM is completed by a healthcare professional for the patient.

## UK FIM + FAM

This scale was developed in the UK, and was last modified by the UK FIM+FAM Group in 1999.[4] Some of the items used in the original FAM from the US Developmental Group in California were considered to be too vague. For this reason the UK version was developed after modification of the original FAM. The UK FIM + FAM Group was coordinated by the Regional Rehabilitation Unit at Northwick Park Hospital, Middlesex, UK.[4] This group has improved the consistency of scoring. The original 30 items and 7 levels remain the same as in the original version.

---

**UK FIM + FAM SCALE**

Self-care
1. Eating
2. Grooming
3. Bathing/showering
4. Dressing upper body
5. Dressing lower body
6. Toileting
7. Swallowing*

Sphincters
1. Bladder management
2. Bowel management

Mobility
1. Transfers: bed/chair/wheelchair
2. Transfers: toilet
3. Transfers: bathtub/shower
4. Transfers: car*
5. Locomotion: walking/wheelchair
6. Locomotion: stairs
7. Community mobility*

---

Communication
1. Expression
2. Comprehension
3. Reading*
4. Writing*
5. Speech intelligibility*

Psychosocial
6. Social interaction
7. Emotional status*
8. Adjustment to limitations*
9. Use of leisure time (replaces employability in original version)*

Cognition
10. Problem solving
11. Memory
12. Orientation*
13. Concentration (replaces attention in original version)*
14. Safety awareness (replaces safety judgement in original version)*

*FAM items

**Seven levels for each item**

| Level | | Description |
|---|---|---|
| 7 | Complete independence | Fully independent |
| 6 | Modified independence | Requiring the use of a device but no physical help |
| 5 | Supervision | Requiring only standby assistance or verbal prompting or help with set-up |
| 4 | Minimal assistance | Requiring incidental hands-on help only (subject performs > 75% of the task) |
| 3 | Moderate assistance | Subject still performs 50–75% of the task |
| 2 | Maximal assistance | Subject provides less than half of the effort (25–49%) |
| 1 | Total assistance | Subject contributes < 25% of the effort or is unable to do the task |

## Scoring principles

- Function is assessed on the basis of direct observation.
- Admission scoring is done within 10 days of admission.
- Discharge scoring is done during the last week before discharge.
- Scoring is done by a multi-disciplinary team member.
- The subject is scored on what they *actually do* on a day-to-day basis, not on what they *could do.*
- Do not leave any score blank.
- Score 1 if the subject does not perform the activity at all, or if no information is available.
- If function is variable, use the lower score.

Reproduced with the permission of L Turner-Stokes from Turner-Stokes L, Nyein K, Turner-Stokes T *et al.* The UK FIM+FAM: development and evaluation. *Clin Rehabil.* 1999; **13:** 277–87.

## REFERENCES

1 Hamilton BB, Granger CV, Sherwin FS *et al.* A uniform national data system for medical rehabilitation. In: Fuhrer MJ, editor. *Rehabilitation Outcomes: analysis and measurement.* Baltimore, MD: Brookes; 1987. pp. 137–47.

2 Stineman MG, Jette A, Fiedler R *et al.* Impairment-specific dimensions within the Functional Independence Measure. *Arch Phys Med Rehabil.* 1997; **78:** 636–43.

3 Hall KM, Mann N, High WM *et al.* Functional measures after traumatic brain injury: ceiling effects of FIM, FIM+FAM, DRS and CIQ. *J Head Trauma Rehabil.* 1996; **11:** 27–39.

4 Turner-Stokes L, Nyein K, Turner-Stokes T *et al.* The UK FIM+FAM: development and evaluation. *Clin Rehabil.* 1999; **13:** 277–87.

## FALLS RISK ASSESSMENT TOOLS

Falls in the elderly represent a complex phenomenon and are rarely due to a single cause. A variety of factors are associated with risk of falling among older adults, including the following:

- ▶ physical factors such as history of previous falls, poor gait or balance, muscle weakness, functional limitation, poor vision, arthritis, postural hypotension, sensory deterioration and neurological disorders
- ▶ pharmaceutical factors – use of medications
- ▶ psychiatric factors – cognitive impairment
- ▶ environmental factors.

  Assessment of falls risk may include the following:
- ▶ use of multi-factorial assessment tools that cover a range of falls risk factors. This could enable screening of high-risk populations and targeting of interventions
- ▶ functional mobility assessments that focus on postural stability, including strength, balance, gait and reaction times.

Effective assessment of fall risk requires a holistic approach, and includes review of many complex and interconnected factors. Falls could be the result of one or more complex and interrelated physiological systems impairments as well as environmental factors. The falls risk increases rapidly with advancing age above 65 years. It is difficult to determine what factors affect balance and contribute to falls, and which factors could be addressed to reduce falls.

### Choice of tool

This is difficult. A variety of tools have been assessed and evaluated for their use in predicting falls risk. Different tools have been used in a variety of settings – for example, in the community, at home, and in long-term or acute care.[1] Some of them have focused on balance and gait assessments, while others have focused on risk factors. Target populations within a given setting have varied in studies – for example, those with cognitive impairment, and studies limited to small samples or recurrent fallers. Few tools have been tested more than once in more than one setting. Therefore no single falls risk assessment tool can be recommended for implementation in all settings.

The choice of tool in a particular clinical context should reflect the purpose for which that tool needs to be applied. For example, the screening of a high-risk population requires a tool that is quick and easy to use, with good sensitivity and specificity. If the aim is to reduce risk, the tool should be reliably able to identify remedial risk factors which would allow for tailoring of interventions. Comprehensive medical assessment of fallers is the focus of the Prevention of Falls Network Europe Group (profane.org.eu).

A systematic review of risk assessment tools for falls in hospitalised patients was published in 2004.[2] The authors concluded that few well-validated tools have been described, and that even the best-validated tool could fail to predict a significant number of falls, as fallers are a heterogenous group.[2] However, a small number of readily detectable risk factors have been repeatedly identified in studies. Perhaps the key is to look for reversible falls risk factors in all patients.[2]

Currently the use of falls risk assessment as part of a multi-factorial approach to the prevention of falls is supported by evidence of a strong association between multiple risk factors and falls, and a significant reduction in falls can be achieved where assessment is combined with tailored interventions.[3]

Some of the tools for assessing risk of falling are described below.

### REFERENCES

1 Scott V, Votova K, Scanlan A *et al*. Multifactorial and functional mobility assessment tools for fall risk among older adults in community, home support, long-term and acute care settings. *Age Ageing*. 2007; **36**: 130–39.

2 Oliver D, Daly F, Martin FC *et al*. Risk factors and risk assessment tools for falls in hospitalised patients: a systematic review. *Age Ageing*. 2004; **33**: 122–30.

3 Gillespie LD, Gillespie WJ, Robertson MC *et al*. Interventions for preventing falls in elderly people (Cochrane Review). In: *Cochrane Database of Systematic Reviews. Issue 4*. Chichester: John Wiley & Sons; 2003.

## THE STRATIFY FALLS RISK ASSESSMENT TOOL

This tool was developed and validated in the UK to predict falls.[1]

### Scoring

The tool contains five clinical risk factors associated with falling, and has a simple scoring system. These factors can be readily assessed by ward nurses based upon their day-to-day observation of patients admitted to hospital. A score range of 0 to 5 is derived by scoring 1 point for each of the five factors. The scoring requires no formal measurements, additional training or equipment.

### Time taken

It takes 1 minute to administer this tool.

### Sensitivity and specificity

The ability of the STRATIFY tool to predict falls had 93% sensitivity and 88% specificity amongst the phase 2 population cohort and 92% sensitivity and 68% specificity amongst the phase 3 cohort population studied.[1] The authors found that this tool has high predictive validity. The tool shows reproducibility with the predictive variables tested in different geriatric settings.

### Clinical application

A score of 2 as a definition of high risk identified 93% of falls.[1] This can allow targeting of strategies to prevent falls of patients on the ward. Thus the STRATIFY falls risk assessment tool may be applicable to many acute elderly patients in hospital.

### Limitations

Falls rather than patients were used as outcomes in the STRATIFY study, and this could inflate the predictive validity. Certain patient characteristics may have greater value in predicting falls. The term 'agitation' could have varying interpretations. A prospective cohort study showed that the STRATIFY tool performed poorly as a predictor of falls in stroke patients.[2]

A STRATIFY tool with some modifications and re-weighting of items has been used and developed in a Canadian hospital setting, where it showed good predictive validity in identifying fallers.[3]

## STRATIFY FALLS RISK ASSESSMENT TOOL

Person's name: ....................................................................

Date of assessment: ...........................................................

Choose **one** of the following options which best describes the person's level of capability when transferring from a bed to chair:

| Answer | Score |
|---|---|
| Unable | 0 |
| Needs major help | 1 |
| Needs minor help | 2 |
| Independent | 3 |

Choose **one** of the following options which best describes the person's level of mobility:

| Answer | Score |
|---|---|
| Immobile | 0 |
| Independent with the aid of a wheelchair | 1 |
| Uses walking aid | 2 |
| Walks with the aid of one person | 2 |
| Independent | 3 |

**Total the transfer and mobility score:** _____

| | | Answer | Score |
|---|---|---|---|
| 1 | Is the combined transfer and mobility score 3 or 4? | Yes | 1 |
| | | No | 0 |
| 2 | Has the person had any falls in the last 3 months? | Yes | 1 |
| | | No | 0 |
| 3 | Is the person visually impaired to the extent that everyday function is affected? | Yes | 1 |
| | | No | 0 |
| 4 | Is the person agitated? | Yes | 1 |
| | | No | 0 |

5 Do you think the person is in need of especially frequent toileting?

| | Answer | Score |
|---|---|---|
| | Yes | 1 |
| | No | 0 |

**Total of questions 1–5** _____

0 = low risk   1 = moderate risk   2 or above = high risk

Developed from Oliver D *et al.* Development and evaluation of evidence-based risk assessment tool (STRATIFY) to predict which elderly inpatients will fall. *BMJ.* 1997; **315**: 1049–53. Reproduced with permission from BMJ Publishing Group.

## REFERENCES

1 Oliver D, Britton M, Seed P *et al.* Development and evaluation of evidence-based risk assessment tool (STRATIFY) to predict which elderly inpatients will fall. *BMJ.* 1997; **315**: 1049–53.

2 Smith J, Forster A, Young J. Use of STRATIFY falls risk assessment in patients recovering from stroke. *Age Ageing.* 2006; **35**: 138–43.

3 Papaioannou A, Parkinson W, Cook R *et al.* Prediction of falls using a risk assessment tool in the acute care setting. *BMC Med.* 2004; **2**: 1–7.

## BALANCE TESTS IN OLDER ADULTS

Maintaining balance requires the interaction of skeletal, neuromuscular and sensory systems. A variety of balance tests have been developed for use at home or in hospital. These can assist older adults who are at risk of falling. Among the many tools that have been published, a review[1] identified the following six balance testing tools as most appropriate for clinical use, as they do not require much equipment or training, they can be administered quickly and they can be applied at home or in clinic:

1   the Berg Balance Scale
2   the Clinical Test of Sensory Interaction and Balance
3   the Functional Reach Test
4   the Tinetti Balance Test
5   the Timed Up and Go Test
6   the Physical Performance Test.

The choice of tool depends upon what aspect of balance is to be measured and what the results will be used for. All of the above tools measure balance during voluntary, self-initiated dynamic movements which are involved in the performance of daily activities. The Tinetti Balance Test and the Timed Up and Go Test also measure balance during gait. The Clinical Test of Sensory Interaction and Balance, the Functional Reach Test and the Timed Up and Go Test measure more narrow aspects of balance. The Functional Reach Test and the Timed Up and Go Test are more sensitive to change over time. The Berg Balance Scale and the Functional Reach Test have more evidence for reliability and validity.[1]

For prediction of falls, only the Berg Balance Scale, the Functional Reach Test and the Tinetti Balance Test have actual cut-off scores which are predictive of falls. Therefore these three tools could be useful when setting objective goals for individual patients. However, as balance requires the interaction of many different systems, use of one tool alone may not predict falls. Even then, among the multiple risk factors, altered balance is the greatest contributor towards falls in the elderly.

### REFERENCE

1 Whitney SL, Poole JL, Cass SP. A review of balance instruments for older adults. *Am J Occup Ther.* 1998; **52**: 666–71.

## BERG BALANCE SCALE

This is one of the most widely used tests of functional mobility and balance. It was specifically designed as a measure of balance for use with older people in clinical settings.[1] It is intended to assess a person's ability to perform several common daily living tasks safely. It assesses ability to maintain positions or perform movements of increasing difficulty, progressing from a sitting position to bilateral stance and then to tandem and single leg stance. The ability to change positions is also assessed.

### Scoring

This balance scale[1] is based on 14 items that are common to daily life activities. The items include both simple mobility tasks (transfers, standing unsupported, sit to stand) and more difficult tasks (tandem standing, turning through 360 degrees, single leg stance). The items are graded on a 5-point ordinal scale from 0 to 4, with a maximum possible score of 56 points. A score of 0 is given if the participant is unable to perform the task, and a score of 4 is given if they are able to do the task.

### Instructions

▶ Please document each task and/or give instructions as written.
▶ When scoring, record the *lowest* response category that applies for each item.
▶ For most items, subjects are asked to maintain a given position for a specific length of time.
▶ Progressively more points are deducted if:
  ● the time or distance requirements are not met
  ● the subject's performance warrants supervision
  ● the subject touches an external support or receives assistance from the examiner.
▶ The subject should understand that they must maintain their balance while attempting the tasks.
▶ The choice of which leg to stand on or how far to reach is left to the subject.
▶ Chairs that are used should be of reasonable height.
▶ Either a stool or a step of average step height should be used for item 12.

| Berg Balance Scale score | Falls risk |
| --- | --- |
| 41–56 | Low |
| 21–40 | Medium |
| 0–20 | High |

Assistive devices cannot be used. However, personal assistance is permitted during the test and is incorporated into the scoring system.

### Administration time
It takes around 15 minutes to administer this tool.

### Tools
A stopwatch, ruler, chair, bed and stool are needed.

### Reliability
The psychometric properties of this tool have been extensively tested. The tool has demonstrated adequate inter-rater (Intraclass Correlation Coefficient (ICC) = 0.98) and high intra-rater (ICC = 0.98) reliability and high internal consistency (Cronbach's alpha coefficient = 0.96).[2]

### Concurrent validity
With the Barthel Index, r = 0.67, with the Timed Up and Go Test, r = –0.76, and with the Tinetti Balance Test, r = 0.91.[3]

### Clinical application
A score of < 45 was shown to be predictive of falls in older adults.[3] However, a later study showed that this cut-off score was only 53% sensitive in identifying people who fall, but was specific in identifying people who do not fall.[4] In other words, older adults who scored higher than a cut-off score of 45 were less likely to fall than those who scored below that cut-off score. The Berg Balance Scale also predicted a person's use of an assistive device,[4] as the scores of people who used a walker or cane indoors were different from each other and lower than those of individuals who only used a cane outdoors, or who walked without an assistive device. The Berg Balance Scale differentiated people with stroke from people without stroke.[4]

Scores can improve after training in mobility and balance, and the test is responsive to changes in clinical status. The Berg Balance Scale measures many aspects of balance, and requires very little equipment.

The scale has been used for insurance reports and the Medicare Program in the USA. In an investigation of the feasibility of using different clinical measures as screening tests for referral to physical therapy, the Berg Balance Scale yielded one of the most promising results.[5]

### Limitations
This scale takes 15 minutes to administer, which is longer than the other balance scales. There is a potential ceiling effect with higher-level patients. The Berg

Balance Scale does not include gait items. Some training is required in the use of the scale.

### Modification

A lower cut-off score of 40/56 has been recommended for assessing fall risk.[6] Although the original scale is used without modifications, it has been recommended that users omit the first 5 items on the scale if the subject is able to stand.[7]

---

**BERG BALANCE SCALE**

Patient's name: .................................................................

Date: ..............................................................................

1. **Sitting to standing**

   Please stand up. Try not to use your hands for support.

   Able to stand, not using hands, and stabilise independently = 4 points

   Able to stand independently using hands = 3 points

   Able to stand using hands after several tries = 2 points

   Needs minimal assistance to stand and stabilise = 1 point

   Needs moderate or maximal assistance to stand = 0 points

2. **Standing unsupported**

   Stand for 2 minutes without holding on to support.

   Able to stand safely for 2 minutes = 4 points

   Able to stand for 2 minutes with supervision = 3 points

   Able to stand for 30 seconds, unsupported = 2 points

   Needs several tries to stand for 30 seconds, unsupported = 1 point

   Unable to stand for 30 seconds, unassisted = 0 points

3. **Sitting unsupported, with feet on floor**

   Sit with arms folded for 2 minutes.

   Able to sit safely and securely for 2 minutes = 4 points

   Able to sit for 2 minutes under supervision = 3 points

   Able to sit for 30 seconds = 2 points

   Able to sit for 10 seconds = 1 point

   Unable to sit unsupported = 0 points

---

4.  **Standing to sitting**

    Please sit down.

    Sits safely with minimal use of hands = 4 points

    Controls descent by using hands = 3 points

    Uses backs of legs against chair to control descent = 2 points

    Sits independently but has uncontrolled descent = 1 point

    Needs assistance to sit down = 0 points

5.  **Transfers**

    Please move from chair to bed and back again.

    One way towards a seat with armrests.

    One way towards a seat without armrests.

    Able to transfer safely with minimal use of hands = 4 points

    Able to transfer safely with definite use of hands = 3 points

    Able to transfer safely with verbal cueing and/or supervision
    = 2 points

    Needs assistance of one person = 1 point

    Needs assistance of two people to transfer safely/unable to
    transfer = 0 points

6.  **Standing unsupported with eyes closed**

    Close your eyes and stand still for 10 seconds.

    Able to stand still for 10 seconds safely = 4 points

    Able to stand still for 10 seconds with supervision = 3 points

    Able to stand still for 3 seconds = 2 points

    Unable to keep eyes closed for 3 seconds, but stays steady =
    1 point

    Needs help to keep from falling = 0 points

7.  **Standing unsupported with feet together**

    Place your feet together and stand without holding on to support.

    Able to place feet together independently and stand safely for
    1 minute = 4 points

    Able to place feet together independently and stand for 1 minute
    with supervision = 3 points

    Able to place feet together independently, but unable to hold for
    30 seconds = 2 points

Needs help to attain position, but able to stand for 15 seconds
= 1 point

Needs help to attain position, and unable to hold for 15 seconds
= 0 points

8. **Reaching forward with outstretched arm**

Lift arms to 90 degrees. Examiner places ruler at the fingertips
when arm is at 90 degrees. Stretch out your fingers and reach
forward as far as you can. Do not move your feet. When possible
use both arms to avoid rotation of trunk.

Can reach forward confidently more than 10 inches = 4 points

Can reach forward more than 5 inches = 3 points

Can reach forward more than 2 inches = 2 points

Reaches forward, but needs supervision = 1 point

Needs help to keep from falling = 0 points

9. **Picking up item from floor**

Pick up the shoe/slipper which is placed in front of you on the floor.

Able to pick up the slipper safely and easily = 4 points

Able to pick up the slipper, but needs supervision, and keeps
balance independently = 3 points

Unable to pick up the slipper, reaches 2–3 inches from it = 2 points

Unable to pick up the slipper, and needs supervision when trying
= 1 point

Unable to pick up the slipper, and needs assistance to keep from
falling = 0 points

10. **Turning to look behind over left and right shoulder**

Turn to look behind you over your left shoulder, and then repeat
over your right shoulder.

Looks behind from both sides and shifts weight well = 4 points

Looks behind to one side only, other side shows less weight shift
= 3 points

Turns sideways only, but maintains balance = 2 points

Needs supervision when turning = 1 point

Needs assistance to keep from falling = 0 points

11. **Turning through 360 degrees**

Turn around completely in a full circle one way, pause, and then turn a full circle in the opposite direction.

Able to turn through 360° safely each way in less than 4 seconds = 4 points

Able to turn through 360° safely to one side in less than 4 seconds = 3 points

Able to turn through 360° safely but slowly = 2 points

Needs close supervision or verbal cueing = 1 point

Needs assistance while turning = 0 points

12. **Number of times stool touched while stepping**

Place each foot alternately on the stool. Continue until each foot has touched the stool four times.

Able to stand independently and safely and complete 8 steps in 20 seconds = 4 points

Able to stand independently and complete 8 steps in 20 seconds = 3 points

Able to complete 4 steps, without aid, with supervision = 2 points

Able to complete more than 2 steps, needs minimal assistance = 1 point

Needs assistance to keep from falling/unable to try = 0 points

13. **Standing unsupported with one foot in front of the other**

(Demonstrate this to subject first.) Place one foot in front of the other. If you feel that you cannot place your foot directly in front, try to step far enough ahead for the heel of your forward foot to be in front of the toes of the other foot.

Able to place feet in tandem independently and hold for 30 seconds = 4 points

Able to place one foot in front of the other independently and hold for 30 seconds = 3 points

Able to take small step independently and hold for 30 seconds = 2 points

Needs help to step, but can hold for 15 seconds = 1 point

Loses balance while stepping or standing = 0 points

14. **Standing on one leg**

Stand on one leg for as long as you can without holding on.

Able to lift leg independently and hold for 10 seconds = 4 points

Able to lift leg independently and hold for 5–10 seconds = 3 points

Able to lift leg for more than 3 seconds = 2 points

Tries to lift leg, unable to hold for 3 seconds, but remains standing independently = 1 point

Unable to try, or needs assistance to prevent falling = 0 points

**Total score (maximum possible score = 56)**

Reproduced with the permission of Dr KO Berg from Berg KO, Wood-Dauphinee SL, Williams JI *et al.* Measuring balance in the elderly: preliminary development of an instrument. *Physiother Can.* 1989; **41**: 304–11.

## REFERENCES

1 Berg KO, Wood-Dauphinee SL, Williams JI *et al.* Measuring balance in the elderly: preliminary development of an instrument. *Physiother Can.* 1989; **41**: 304–11.

2 Berg KO, Wood-Dauphinee SL, Williams JI. The balance scale: reliability assessment with elderly residents and patients with an acute stroke. *Scand J Rehabil Med.* 1995; **27**: 27–36.

3 Berg KO, Maki BE, Williams JI *et al.* Clinical and laboratory measures of postural balance in an elderly population. *Arch Phys Med Rehabil.* 1992; **73**: 1073–80.

4 Thorbahn LDB, Newton RA. Use of the Berg balance test to predict falls in elderly persons. *Phys Ther.* 1996; **76**: 576–83.

5 Harada N, Chiu V, Damron-Rodriguez J *et al.* Screening for balance and mobility impairment in elderly individuals living in residential care facilities. *Phys Ther.* 1995; **75**: 462–9.

6 Riddle DL, Startford PW. Interpreting validity indexes for diagnostic tests: an illustration using the Berg balance test. *Phys Ther.* 1999; **79**: 939–48.

7 Newton R. Balance screening of an inner-city older adult population. *Arch Phys Med Rehabil.* 1997; **78**: 587–91.

## FUNCTIONAL REACH TEST

Functional reach manoeuvres have been used extensively by the US Department of Transportation, the National Aeronautics and Space Administration (NASA)

and the US Automotive Industry for safety and functional utility of vehicle design. For older adults, functional reach is a dynamic measure of stability during a self-initiated movement.[1] The Functional Reach Test was designed as a clinical measure of balance, and was originally tested on a sample of 128 community-dwelling adults between 21 and 87 years of age.[1]

### Scoring

Functional reach is the difference in inches between a person's arm length and maximum forward reach with the shoulder flexed to 90 degrees while maintaining a fixed base of support in standing. In other words, it is the maximum distance one can reach forward beyond arm's length. The distance is measured with a yardstick mounted on the wall, parallel to the floor, at the level of the person's shoulder.

The subject is asked to stand with their feet a comfortable distance apart, to make a fist and to forward flex the dominant arm to approximately 90 degrees. They are then asked to reach forward as far as possible without taking a step or touching the wall. The distance between the start and end points is measured using the head of the metacarpal of the third finger as the reference point.[1] Two practice trials and three test trials are performed, with the mean of the three test trials documented in inches or centimetres. A carefully trained clinician should be capable of reading the measurement on a yardstick to the nearest 0.5 inches.

### FUNCTIONAL REACH NORMS

| Age (years) | Men (inches) | Women (inches) |
|---|---|---|
| 20–40 | 16.7±1.9 | 14.6±2.2 |
| 41–69 | 14.9±2.2 | 13.8±2.2 |
| 70–87 | 13.2±1.6 | 10.5±3.5 |

Reproduced with the permission of the Gerontological Society of America from Duncan PW, Weiner DK, Chandler J *et al.* Functional reach: a new clinical measure of balance. *J Gerontol.* 1990; **45**: M195.

### Administration time

It takes 1–2 minutes to administer the test.

### Tools

A yardstick, Velcro and level are needed.

### Reliability

The test has good inter-rater reliability (ICC = 0.98) and test–retest reliability (r = 0.89).[2]

### Concurrent validity

This has been determined with walking speed (r = 0.71), tandem walk (r = 0.71) and mobility skills (r = 0.65).[2]

### Clinical application

A score of ≤ 6 was shown to be predictive of falls in the elderly[3] (predictive validity). The Functional Reach Test measures dynamic postural control. It is a continuous measurement system that enables greater sensitivity than categorical or ordinal measures. The advantages of functional reach are that it is a quick, precise and portable test, it requires minimum equipment, is single task and is sensitive to change following balance training.

### Limitations

The test measures dynamic stability in only one direction and with no change in the base of support. Many activities that are difficult for the elderly, such as gait, involve controlled movement of the centre of mass laterally as well as in an anterior direction and outside the stability limits. Height, age and gender can influence the results to a certain extent. It is difficult to perform the Functional Reach Test in patients with dementia or spinal deformities, and in frail individuals who are unable to stand unsupported. Also it can only be used to test individuals who have adequate shoulder range of motion to perform the test and are able to maintain a standing position for several minutes without an assistive device.

Despite its limitations, this test is a useful tool for screening, assessing, monitoring over time and even predicting functional status in older people. It is appropriate in a variety of settings, including acute care, inpatient and outpatient rehabilitation, home health and community screening.

The test has been expanded to include reaching to both sides and behind the subject.[4]

## Lateral Reach Test

This test was developed to assess mediolateral postural control.[5] The subject stands near a wall with their arm abducted at 90 degrees. They are asked to reach directly sideways as far as possible without overbalancing, moving step or touching a wall. No knee flexion or trunk rotation is permitted. Maximum hand excursion is measured. In a study of 60 community–dwelling women aged 72.5±5 years, the mean lateral reach observed was 20.0±4.88 cm, with a range of 10–36 cm.[5] The test–retest reliability was very high (ICC = 0.943). The results decrease with increasing age, decreasing height and decreasing arm length.

## REFERENCES

1 Duncan PW, Weiner DK, Chandler J *et al.* Functional reach: a new clinical measure of balance. *J Gerontol.* 1990; **45**: M192–7.

2 Weiner DK, Bongiorni DR, Studenski SA *et al.* Does functional reach improve with rehabilitation? *Arch Phys Med Rehabil.* 1993; **74**: 796–800.

3 Duncan PW, Studenski S, Chandler J *et al.* Functional reach: predictive validity in a sample of elderly male veterans. *J Gerontol.* 1992; **47**: M93–8.

4 Newton R. Reach in four directions as a measure of stability in older adults. *Phys Ther.* 1996; **76**: S23.

5 Brauer S, Burns Y, Galley P. Lateral reach. A clinical measure of medio–lateral postural stability. *Physiother Res Int.* 1999; **4**: 81–8.

## TINETTI BALANCE TEST

This is a performance test of balance and gait during manoeuvres used during normal daily activities.[1]

### *Scoring*

Scoring is done on a 3-point ordinal scale with a range of 0–2, where a score of 0 represents maximum impairment and a score of 2 represents independence. The individual scores are then combined to form three measures – *gait score*, *balance score* and *overall score*. The test has two components.

▶ *The balance portion* has 9 manoeuvres which are graded on an ordinal scale as either normal adaptive or abnormal. The maximum total score is 16 points.

▶ *The gait portion* has 7 gait characteristics which are graded as normal or abnormal. The maximum total score is 12 points. The subject first walks at 'usual pace' and then walks at 'rapid but safe pace.'

The total mobility score for balance and gait is then calculated. The maximum possible score is 28 points.

| Tinetti total score | Risk of falls |
|---|---|
| ≤ 18 | High |
| 19–23 | Moderate |
| ≥ 24 | Low |

### Administration time

It takes around 10 minutes to administer the test.

### Tools

A chair, stopwatch, 5 lb object and 15-foot walkway are required.

### Reliability

The inter-rater reliability is 85%.[2]

### Concurrent validity

With the Berg scale, r = 0.91, with stride length r = 0.62–0.68, and with single leg stance r = 0.59–0.64.[2]

### Clinical application

Four items related to balance (unsteady sitting down, unable to stand in single stance, unsteady turning, and unsteady when nudged) and three items related to gait (increased trunk sway, increased path deviation, and speed) in combination have been found to predict falls.[3] People with scores of < 18 have an increased risk of falls for balance and gait items.[4] Scores can improve after training on gait and balance items. The advantages of the Tinetti Balance Test are that it assesses many aspects of balance, and is simple and quick to use, but it is not sensitive enough to changes in balance.

---

**TINETTI ASSESSMENT TOOL: BALANCE**

Patient's name: ..................................... Date: ...........

Location: ........................................... Rater: ..........

.............................................................

Initial instructions: The subject is seated on a hard, armless chair. The following manoeuvres are tested.

| Task | Description of balance | Possible points | Score |
|------|------------------------|-----------------|-------|
| 1. Sitting balance | Leans or slides in chair | 0 | |
| | Steady and safe | 1 | |
| 2. Arises | Unable to arise without help | 0 | |
| | Able to arise, uses arms to help | 1 | |
| | Able to arise without using arms | 2 | |

---

| Task | Description of balance | Possible points | Score |
|------|------------------------|-----------------|-------|
| 3. Attempts to arise | Unable to attempt to arise without help | 0 | |
| | Able to arise, requires more than one attempt | 1 | |
| | Able to arise in one attempt | 2 | |
| 4. Immediate standing balance (first 5 seconds) | Unsteady (swaggers, moves feet, trunk sway) | 0 | |
| | Steady, but uses walker or other support | 1 | |
| | Steady without walker or other support | 2 | |
| 5. Standing balance | Unsteady | 0 | |
| | Steady, but wide stance (medial heels > 4 inches apart), and uses cane or other support | 1 | |
| | Narrow stance without support | 2 | |
| 6. Nudged (subject at maximum position with feet as close together as possible, examiner pushes lightly on subject's sternum with palm of hand three times) | Begins to fall | 0 | |
| | Staggers, grabs, catches self | 1 | |
| | Steady | 2 | |
| 7. Eyes closed (at maximum position no. 6) | Unsteady | 0 | |
| | Steady | 1 | |
| 8. Turning through 360 degrees | Discontinuous steps | 0 | |
| | Continuous steps | 1 | |
| | Unsteady (grabs, staggers) | 0 | |
| | Steady | 1 | |
| 9. Sitting down | Unsafe (misjudged distance, falls into chair) | 0 | |
| | Uses arms or not a smooth motion | 1 | |
| | Safe, smooth motion | 2 | |
| | **Balance score (out of 16):** | | |

## TINETTI ASSESSMENT TOOL: GAIT

Patient's name: ........................................ Date: ...........

Location: ........................................... Rater: ..........

.................................................

Initial instructions: Subject stands with examiner, walks halfway down or across the room, first at 'usual' pace, then back at 'rapid but safe' pace (using usual walking aids).

| Task | Description of balance | Possible points | Score |
|------|------------------------|-----------------|-------|
| 10. Initiation of gait (immediately after subject is told to 'go') | Any hesitancy or multiple attempts to start | 0 | |
| | No hesitancy | 1 | |
| 11. Step length and height | Right swing foot does not pass left stance foot with step | 0 | |
| | Right foot passes left stance foot | 1 | |
| | Right foot does not clear the floor completely with step | 0 | |
| | Right foot completely clears floor | 1 | |
| | Left swing foot does not pass right stance foot with step | 0 | |
| | Left foot passes right foot stance | 1 | |
| | Left foot does not clear floor completely with step | 0 | |
| | Left foot completely clears floor | 1 | |
| 12. Step symmetry | Right and left step length not equal | 0 | |
| | Right and left step appear equal | 1 | |
| 13. Step continuity | Stopping or discontinuity between steps | 0 | |
| | Steps appear continuous | 1 | |

82

| Task | Description of balance | Possible points | Score |
|------|------------------------|-----------------|-------|
| 14. Path (estimated in relation to floor tiles 12 inches in diameter; observe excursion of 1 foot over about 10 feet of the course) | Marked deviation | 0 | |
| | Mild/moderate deviation or uses walking aid | 1 | |
| | Straight without walking aid | 2 | |
| 15. Trunk | Marked sway or uses walking aid | 0 | |
| | No sway, but flexion of knees or back, or spreads arms out while walking | 1 | |
| | No sway, no flexion, no use of arms, and no use of walking aid | 2 | |
| 16. Walking stance | Heels apart | 0 | |
| | Heels almost touching while walking | 1 | |
| | **Gait score (out of 12):** | | |
| | **Balance and gait score (out of 28):** | | |

Reproduced with the permission of Mary Tinetti from Tinetti ME. Performance-oriented assessment of mobility problems in elderly patients. *J Am Geriatr Soc.* 1986; **34:** 119–26.

## REFERENCES

1 Tinetti ME. Performance-oriented assessment of mobility problems in elderly patients. *J Am Geriatr Soc.* 1986; **34:** 119–26.
2 Berg KO, Maki BE, Williams JI *et al.* Clinical and laboratory measures of postural balance in an elderly population. *Arch Phys Med Rehabil.* 1992; **73:** 1073–80.
3 Tinetti ME, Speechley M, Ginter SF. Risk factors for falls among elderly persons living in the community. *NEJM.* 1988; **319:** 1701–7.
4 Lewis C. Balance gait test proves simple yet useful. *Phys Ther Bull.* 1993; **32:** 40.

## 'TURN 180' TEST

This test is a measure of dynamic postural stability and is designed for use in frail elderly people.[1]

### Scoring

The subject is seated and the procedure is described to them. The subject is then allowed to stand up with or without the help of furniture or other support, with the observer standing behind them. The subject puts their hands by their sides and steps through 180 degrees until they are facing the observer ('Step around until you are facing me'). It is not a timed test, so speed is not important. Count the number of 'finished steps.' Record the direction (clockwise or anticlockwise) and the number of steps taken to complete the 180 degrees turn. The direction of turning does not usually influence the number of steps. Patients with Parkinson's disease could take 18 to 20 steps, patients with with painful knees could take 6 steps, and most elderly people take about 4 steps.[1]

### Reliability

Retest reliability is good.[1] The test has been found to have significant correlations with walking speed, falling history and perceived steadiness.[1]

### Clinical application

The test is simple to use, and clinically useful, especially in the elderly. It is quick to administer, easy for both patient and operator, and no expensive technology is required. It is useful in both community and hospital settings. In one study, community-dwelling elderly who had fallen previously and who took 5 or more steps to complete the turn had an unadjusted risk of 1.9 of sustaining two or more falls during a 1-year follow-up.[2]

### REFERENCES

1 Simpson JM, Worsfold C, Reilly E *et al*. A standard procedure for using TURN 180: testing dynamic postural stability among elderly people. *Physiotherapy*. 2002; **88**: 342–53.

2 Nevitt MC, Cummings SR, Kidd S *et al*. Risk factors for non-syncopal falls. *JAMA*. 1989; **261**: 2663–8.

## 360-DEGREE TURN

This is the number of steps counted when the subject turns through 360 degrees.[1] In one study a sample of 199 elderly people aged 55–70 years were tested in their own homes on two occasions, with good reliability (ICC = 0.92) and better than walking speed test (ICC = 0.78).[1] Another study found that among elderly people living in a care home, 66% of those who fell took more than 12 steps to complete a turn, whereas only 23% of individuals who did not fall needed to take so many steps.[2]

### REFERENCES

1 Tager IB, Swanson A, Satariano WA. Reliability of physical performance measures and self-reported functional measures in an older population. *J Gerontol.* 1998; **53**: M295–300.

2 Lipsitz LA, Jonsson PV, Kelley MM *et al.* Causes and correlates of recurrent falls in ambulatory frail elderly. *J Gerontol.* 1991; **46**: M114–22.

## OTHER SIMPLE BALANCE TESTS THAT ARE USEFUL IN A BUSY CLINICAL SETTING

Some other simple tests for risk assessment of fallers include the following:

1 Chair Stand Test – time taken to stand up and sit down 5 times with the arms crossed.[1]

2 Tandem Walk Test – walking heel to toe in a straight line.[2] Also the Semi-Tandem Stand Test and the Side by Side Stand Test.

3 Foot Tapping Test – time taken to tap one foot back and forth 10 times between two circles placed 30 cm apart in a sitting position.[2]

4 Leg extensor power.[3]

5 Body sway as a measure of postural stability.[4]

### REFERENCES

1 Cummings SR, Nevitt MC, Browner WC *et al.* Risk factors for hip fracture in white women. *NEJM.* 1995; **332**: 767–73.

2 Dargent-Molina P, Favier F, Grandjean M *et al.* Fall-related factors and risk of hip fracture: the EPIDOS prospective study. *Lancet.* 1996; **348**: 145–9.

3 Bassey EJ, Fiatarone MA, O Neil EF *et al.* Leg extensor power and functional performance in very old men and women. *Clin Sci.* 1992; **82**: 321–7.

4 Lord SR, Clark RD, Webster IW. Physiological factors associated with falls in an elderly population. *J Am Geriatr Soc.* 1991; **39**: 1194–200.

## FUNCTIONAL MOBILITY TESTS: TIMED WALKING TESTS

The time taken by a person to walk a certain set distance can be measured. Timed measures may be:

1 distance related – time taken to cover 2 to 20 metres. In practice, the time taken to cover 10 metres is more easily understood.
2 time related – the distance covered over a period of 2 to 12 minutes.

Measurement of gait speed by using timed walking tests can be easily accomplished in clinic or in the subjects's home. The tests are quick and simple to use, and the only equipment needed is a stopwatch and tape measure. Gait speed is useful as an outcome measure in studies of balance and locomotion during rehabilitation after stroke.[1] The test results correlate with recovery after stroke.[2] Reliability has been tested in hospital settings in patients up to 6 months following stroke,[3] and in patients at home 2 years following stroke.[4] High inter-class correlations have been reported of intra- and inter-assessment reliability of gait speeds.[3]

### 10-metre timed walk

This is a measure of self-selected walking speed.

### *Scoring*

This involves asking the subject to walk a set distance, such as 5 metres and then returning, or 10 metres.[5] The walking distance is measured with a metal tape measure and marked with tape on the floor. Five extra metres both ahead and at the end of the 10-metre distance are measured and marked to allow the subject enough distance to accelerate and decelerate. The subject is instructed to 'walk at your normal comfortable pace using any customary walking aids.' The tester times the 10-metre walk to the nearest one-hundredth of a second using a digital stopwatch. Timing begins when the subject crosses the start line, and ends when the leading foot crosses the finish line. The subject performs one practice trial and two test trials, and the latter are averaged to determine self-selected gait velocity.[6] Self-selected gait velocity is a continuous measure recorded in metres/second and obtained by dividing the 10-metre distance walked by the time required to complete that distance. Active community-dwelling older adults have average walking speeds of 0.9 to 1.2 metres/second, and unaided gait in ambulatory nursing home residents averages 0.5 metres/second.[7]

### *Validity and reliability*

This measure is valid and sensitive to change. It has high test–retest and inter-observer reliability.[8] Floor and ceiling effects are minimal in the ambulatory population over 65 years of age.

### Clinical applications

This is a simple, reliable and practically useful test that requires minimum equipment and is useful in domiciliary settings as well, as a maximum 5-metres walk within a house can be assessed.

Usually a 10-metre timed walk is used in practice. For patients with Parkinson's disease, a 20-metre walk can be used. The results can be recorded and easily communicable. The use of aids during the walk should be recorded. This test has been used to make decisions about mobility allowance in the UK.

## Get Up and Go Test

This is a performance-based measure involving multiple tasks.[9] The test requires the subject to rise from a chair, walk 3 metres, turn around, walk back to the chair and sit down. It is scored as follows:

▶ normal, 1 point
▶ very slightly abnormal, 2 points
▶ mildly abnormal, 3 points
▶ moderately abnormal, 4 points
▶ severely abnormal, 5 points.

An increased risk of falls is seen in elderly individuals with a score of ≥ 3. The test standardises most of the basic mobility manoeuvres, and is quick and practical to use. However, the scoring is imprecise. Scoring of performance is rated on a scale of 1 to 5 according to the observer's perception of the patient's risk of falling. The extremes of the scale, 1 and 5, are easy to score, but the intermediate grades are less clear. Thus variation in scores could occur with different observers.

## Timed Up and Go Test

This is similar to the Get Up and Go Test, except for the scoring.[10] It evaluates basic mobility skills in older adults. The Timed Up and Go Test is simply the amount of time taken to do the whole test. The test is quick, requires no special equipment, and can easily be done during a routine medical evaluation. The test can quantify functional mobility, and this may be useful when following clinical change over time. Furthermore, it predicts the patient's ability to go outside alone safely.

### Scoring

A standard armchair is used with a seat height of 46 cm. The subject wears their normal footwear and uses their customary walking aid. No physical assistance is provided. Instructions are given to the subject. On the word 'go', the subject is to get up, walk at their self-selected 'comfortable and safe pace' to a line on the floor 3 metres away, turn and then return to the chair again. The tester uses a digital stopwatch to measure the time to the nearest one-hundredth of a second. The subject performs one practice trial and two test trials, and the latter are averaged to obtain a measure which is recorded in seconds.[10] A neurologically intact, independently mobile adult is able to perform the test in less than 10 seconds.

### Administration time
The test takes 1 to 2 minutes to administer.

### Tools
A chair, a 3-metre walkway and a stopwatch are needed.

### Reliability
The test has high inter-rater reliability (r = 0.99), high intra-rater reliability (r = 0.99) and good retest reliability in different settings.[11]

### Validity
The test has content validity – that is, it evaluates a well-recognised series of manoeuvres used in daily life. It also has concurrent validity[10] – that is, it correlates closely with more extensive measures of balance, gait speed and functional abilities, such as the Berg Balance Scale (r = –0.81), gait speed (r = –0.61) and the Barthel Index of ADL (r = –0.78).

### Clinical application
The Timed Up and Go Test can be used as a screening test or as a descriptive test.[10] If it is used as a screening test, the time score indicates the patient's level of physical mobility. It can discriminate between the freely independent individuals who can perform the test in less than 10 seconds, as compared with very dependent subjects who cannot transfer out of the chair. For those patients who fall between these two extremes the time score also indicates balance, gait, speed and functional capacity. The healthcare professional can then focus on the areas that require further assessment, bypassing irrelevant tests. As a descriptive tool the time score describes the subject's balance, gait speed and level of functional capacity. It is also possible to ascertain from a telephone description the difficulties in balance, transfers, walking outside and climbing stairs.[10]

This test has been shown to be an independent predictor of nursing home placement.[12] The test has shown an independent association, with increased risk of falls.[13] Failure to complete the 5-metre Timed Up and Go Test in 30 seconds was found to be associated with a threefold increased risk of future falling.[14] A cut-off of 12 seconds for the 3-metre version of the Timed Up and Go Test has been suggested as a screening tool for making a further in-depth mobility assessment, rather than as a predictor of falls.[15]

The measure is simple and quick to administer, can be performed by non-professional staff, and does not require much equipment. It can be useful in many different clinical settings, provided that the subject is able to transfer and walk short distances without personal assistance. It may not offer sufficient challenge for assessment of healthy community-dwelling older adults.

### Limitation

Only a few aspects of balance, such as rising, walking and turning, are tested.

## Six-Minute Walking Test

This test measures the maximum distance that a person can walk in 6 minutes. The test is a modification of the Twelve-Minute Walk-Run Test originally developed by Cooper[16] to predict maximum oxygen uptake. The Six-Minute Walking Test has been used to assess function in patients with cardiovascular or pulmonary diseases.[17] Walking a distance of less than 300 metres in 6 minutes predicted increased likelihood of dying in patients with left ventricular dysfunction.[18] Gender-specific regression equations have been developed for adults without known pathology, based on age, weight and height.[19]

### REFERENCES

1 Wade DT, Wood VA, Heller A *et al.* Walking after stroke: measurement and recovery over the first 3 months. *Scand J Rehabil Med.* 1987; **19**: 25–30.

2 Brandstater ME, de Bruin H, Gowland C *et al.* Hemiplegic gait: analysis of temporal variables. *Arch Phys Med Rehabil.* 1983; **64**: 583–7.

3 Hill KD, Goldie PA, Baker PA *et al.* Retest reliability of the temporal and distance characteristics of hemiplegic gait using a footswitch system. *Arch Phys Med Rehabil.* 1994; **75**: 577–83.

4 Collen FM, Wade DT, Bradshaw CM. Mobility after stroke: reliability of measures of impairment and disability. *Int Disabil Stud.* 1990; **12**: 6–9.

5 Kressig RW, Wolff SL, Sattin RW *et al.* Associations of demographic, functional and behavioural characteristics with activity-related fear of falling among older adults transitioning to frailty. *J Am Geriatr Soc.* 2001; **49**: 1456–62.

6 Purser J. *Measures of disability-related outcomes in the clinical setting: practical issues in administration of measures.* Paper presented at Annual Meeting of the American

Geriatrics Society and the American Federation for Aging Research, Duke University Medical Center, Center for Study of Aging and Human Development, Durham, NC, 2 May 1996.

7 Bohannon R, Andrews A, Thomas M. Walking speed: reference values and correlates for older adults. *J Orthop Sports Phys Ther.* 1996; **24**: 86–90.

8 Wade DT, Langton HR. Functional abilities after stroke: measurement, natural history and prognosis. *J Neurol Neurosurg Psychiatry.* 1987; **50**: 177–82.

9 Mathias S, Nayak USL, Issacs B. Balance in elderly patients. The 'get up and go' test. *Arch Phys Med Rehabil.* 1986; **67**: 387–9.

10 Podsiadlo D, Richardson S. The timed 'up and go': a test of basic functional mobility for frail elderly persons. *J Am Geriatr Soc.* 1991; **39**: 142–8.

11 Morris S, Morris ME, Lansek R. Reliability of measurements obtained with the timed 'up and go' test in people with Parkinson's disease. *Phys Ther.* 2001; **81**: 810–18.

12 Nikolaus T, Bach M, Oster P *et al.* Prospective value of self-report and performance-based tests of functional status for 18-month outcomes in elderly patients. *Aging (Milano).* 1996; **8**: 271–6.

13 Shumway-Cook A, Brauer S, Woollacott M. Predicting the probability for falls in community-dwelling older adults using the Timed Up and Go Test. *Phys Ther.* 2000; **80**: 896–903.

14 Morris R, Harwood R, Baker R *et al.* A comparison of different balance tests in the prediction of falls in older women with vertebral fractures: a cohort study. *Age Ageing.* 2007; **36**: 78–83.

15 Bischoff HA, Stahelin HB, Monsch AU *et al.* Identifying a cut-off point for normal mobility: a comparison of the timed 'up and go' test in community-dwelling and institutionalised elderly women. *Age Ageing.* 2003; **32**: 315–20.

16 Cooper KH. A means of assessing maximal oxygen uptake: correlation between field and treadmill testing. *JAMA.* 1968: **203**: 201–4.

17 Swisher A, GoldfarbA. Use of the six-minute walk/run test to predict peak oxygen consumption in older adults. *Cardiopulm Phys Ther.* 1998; **9**: 3–5.

18 Bittner V, Weiner DH, Yusuf S *et al.* Prediction of mortality and morbidity with a six-minute walk test in patients with left ventricular dysfunction. *Rehabil Nurs.* 1997; **22**: 177–81.

19 Enright PL, Sherill DL. Reference equations for the six-minute walk in healthy adults. *Am J Respir Crit Care Med.* 1998; **158**: 1384–7.

## Three-Minute Walking Test

This is a quick and easy gait test for clinical use. It was originally developed to assess functional gait in patients with neurological dysfunction.[1] The subject is asked to walk a predetermined course at a comfortable, self-selected pace using whatever assistive device is normally chosen when walking outside the home. The subject is allowed to rest, but the clock continues to run during any rest stops. The following items are measured:

▶ heart rate before and after the walk
▶ distance covered
▶ number of stops
▶ number of deviations from the 15-inch-wide path.

After the subject has completed the test, the clinician notes the total distance travelled in 3 minutes. An average older adult without any neurological impairment can walk about 727±148 feet in 3 minutes (73 metres/minute), compared with 323±166 feet (32 metres/minute) for a group that includes fallers.[1] For a person to be considered ambulatory in the community, they should be able to walk about 330 feet in 3 minutes.

### REFERENCE

1 Shumway-Cook A, Woollacott MH. *Motor Control: theory and practical applications.* Philadelphia, PA: Lippincott, Williams and Wilkins; 2001.

## STANDARDISED GAIT SCORING AND
## INSTRUMENTED GAIT ANALYSIS

Gait assessment is important for managing gait problems. A variety of methods are used by researchers for scoring gait analysis for gait impairments. Walking time, stride length, step length asymmetry, velocity, balance, arm swing, etc. using videos and computer-assisted programs have been used as variables to assess gait characteristics. However, there is no uniform single scale in common clinical usage. In a survey of 1826 physiotherapists in the UK National Health Service, it was found that there was no uniform systematic use of standardised gait assessment tools, and only 23% of respondents had patients assessed in a gait laboratory, even though management of abnormal gait constitutes a major aspect of physiotherapy practice.[1]

In their combined guidelines for falls prevention,[2] the American Geriatrics Society and the British Geriatrics Society recommended that all older people who report a fall should be observed with the Get Up and Go Test,[3,4] and those who demonstrate unsteadiness when performing the test require further assessment.

### REFERENCES

1 Toro B, Nester CJ, Farren PC. The status of gait assessment among physiotherapists in the United Kingdom. *Arch Phys Med Rehabil.* 2003; **84**: 1878–84.

2 Panel on Falls Prevention. Guideline for prevention of falls in older persons by American Geriatrics Society, British Geriatrics Society and American Academy of Orthopaedic Surgeons Panel on Falls Prevention. *J Am Geriatr Soc.* 2001; **49**: 664–72.

3 Mathias S, Nayak USL, Issacs B. Balance in elderly patients. The Get Up and Go Test. *Arch Phys Med Rehabil.* 1986; **67**: 387–9.

4 Podsiadlo D, Richardson S. The Timed Up and Go: a test of basic functional mobility for frail elderly persons. *J Am Geriatr Soc.* 1991; **39**: 142–8.

## SCALES USED IN STROKE

Stroke is a difficult disease to study because clinical manifestations are highly variable, there are several causes, and the extent of recovery is variable. Moreover, recovery is difficult to measure quantitatively because traditional neurological examination is suited to accurate description of a single patient, but is ill suited to group description over time, as is required for large-scale clinical investigation trials.[1] Use of proper stroke scales is important for assessment of patients with stroke in both acute and recovery phases, for evaluation of published research, and for selection of appropriate outcome measures for intervention trials. Some of the major issues related to stroke which can be measured include communication, neurological deficit (e.g. hemiparesis), loss of ability to perform specific tasks (e.g. feeding or walking), and loss of ability to function in normal roles (e.g. employment and quality of life). Various tools exist and have been used inconsistently in trials. No single measure can fully describe or predict all dimensions of stroke disability and recovery. Despite these limitations in measuring outcomes, a variety of measurement scales have been used in stroke trials and studies.

In general, data about a particular disease can be classified into one of the following four categories:[2]

1 nominal – based on category (e.g. stroke subtypes classification)
2 ordinal – based upon ranking into one of several ordered states (e.g. measuring motor performance as absent, poor or normal)
3 interval level – based on the difference between two numerical scores (e.g. temperature in Fahrenheit)
4 ratio level – compared with an absolute origin (e.g. height or weight).

All of the measurement scales that are used to assess stroke can be included under any one of the following three categories:[1]

1 global outcome scales – these provide a broad overview and a limited number of discrete categories
2 physical deficit scales – these attach numbers to specific findings on detailed neurological examination
3 ADL scales – these measure aspects of functional recovery using common skills needed for functional independence.

### Global outcome scales

The patient is assigned to a limited number of broad classifications. These scales are simple and easy to use, but there may be lack of standard demarcation between categories.[3] Global rankings lack sensitivity (i.e. power to detect small changes in neurodeficit). Examples include the following:

▶ the Rankin Handicap Scale (*see* page 53)
▶ the Modified Rankin Scale (*see* page 54)
▶ the Glasgow Outcome Scale[4] has been used in studies of outcome following head injury. It has five outcomes, namely death, persistent vegetative state, severe disability, moderate disability and good recovery. This scale is little used in stroke studies
▶ the Stroke Impact Scale[5] – not much used
▶ the Short Form 36[6] (*see* page 118).

## Physical deficit scales

These scales describe stroke-related deficits based on neurological examination. The data are recorded numerically. Examples include the following:

▶ the Mathew Stroke Scale, first published in 1972[7] – an 100-point scale
▶ the National Institutes of Health Stroke Scale[8] (*see* page 97)
▶ the Toronto Stroke Scale, first published in 1976[9] – a 317-point and 11-category scale
▶ the Canadian Neurological Scale, first published in 1986,[10] – a 10-point scale
▶ the Hemispheric Stroke Scale[11] – an 100-point scale
▶ the Scandinavian Stroke Scale.[12]

## ADL scales

These scales measure performance in occupational functions which are essential for independent living. The ADL scales are administered either through patient interview, observation or self-assessment. The functions that are included may be basic (e.g. continence) or more complex (e.g. cooking). These scales are not useful in acute stroke, but are more relevant in rehabilitation settings. Examples include the following:

▶ the Barthel Index (*see* page 42) – a widely used 100-point, 10-item scale
▶ the Nottingham Extended Activities of Daily Living Questionnaire (*see* page 50)
▶ the Kenny Self-Care Evaluation[13] – measures 6 items and 24 points
▶ the Katz Index of Activities of Daily Living[14] – contains 6 rankings in subsequent version
▶ the Activity Index[15] – includes 4 mental capacity items, 6 measures of motor function and 5 measures of ADL.

## Clinical application of stroke scales

The application of valid and reliable standardised stroke scales is necessary in clinical trials conducted in stroke populations in order to accurately quantify progress and recovery. A critical appraisal of stroke rating scales has suggested that clinical stroke trials should include a physical deficit scale and a global rating during the acute phase, and that an ADL scale should be added later during recovery.[1] In a literature review using the Medline search system, which included 21 studies on stroke scales, the authors[16] found that the National Institutes of Health Stroke Scale (NIHSS), the Canadian Neurological Scale and the European Stroke Scale had the highest reliability across items, and the Barthel Index was the most reliable disability scale.

To summarise, some of the most widely used scales include the NIHSS, the Modified Rankin Scale and the Barthel Index. Scales that measure neurological deficit or specific body function are useful early in acute stroke for triage and treatment decisions such as thrombolysis.[17] For example, the NIHSS is valuable for initial assessment of patients with acute stroke in the pre-hospital, emergency department and hospital settings, and moreover it predicts long-term outcomes.[18] The NIHSS can be useful for early prognostication and serial assessment. The Modified Rankin Scale and the Barthel Index are commonly used to assess disability components such as activity and dependency after stroke, and are useful for guiding rehabilitation interventions.

## REFERENCES

1 Lyden PD, Lau GT. A critical appraisal of stroke evaluation and rating scales. *Stroke.* 1991; **22**: 1345–52.

2 Munsat TL. *Quantification of Neurological Deficit.* Boston, MA: Butterworths; 1989.

3 Feinstein AR. *Clinimetrics.* New Haven, CT: Yale University Press; 1987.

4 Jennett B, Bond M. Assessment of outcome after severe brain damage: a practical scale. *Lancet.* 1975; **1**: 480–84.

5 Duncan PW, Bode RK, Min Lai S *et al.* for the Glycine Antagonist in Neuroprotection (GAIN) Americas Investigators. Rasch analysis of a new stroke-specific outcome scale: the Stroke Impact Scale. *Arch Phys Med Rehabil.* 2003; **84**: 950–63.

6 Duncan PW, Jorgensen HS, Wade DT. Outcome measures in acute stroke trials: a systematic review and some recommendations to improve practice. *Stroke.* 2000; **31**: 1429–38.

7 Mathew NT, Rivera VM, Meyer JJ *et al.* Double-blind evaluation of glycerol therapy in acute cerebral infarction. *Lancet.* 1972; **2**: 1327–9.

8 Brott T, Adams HP, Olinger CP *et al.* Measurements of acute cerebral infarction: a clinical examination scale. *Stroke.* 1989; **20**: 864–70.

9 Norris JW. Study design of stroke treatments (letter). *Stroke.* 1982; **13**: 527–8.

10 Cote R, Hatchinski VC, Shurell BL *et al.* The Canadian Neurological Scale: a preliminary study in acute stroke. *Stroke.* 1986; **17**: 731–7.

11 Adams RJ, Meador KJ, Sethi KD *et al.* Graded neurologic scale for use in acute hemispheric stroke treatment protocols. *Stroke.* 1987; **18**: 665–9.

12 Christensen H, Boysen G, Trueben T. The Scandinavian Stroke Scale predicts outcome in patients with mild ischaemic stroke. *Cerebrovasc Dis.* 2005; **20**: 46–8.

13 Schoening HA, Anderegg L, Bergstrom D *et al.* Numerical scoring of self-care status of patients. *Arch Phys Med Rehabil.* 1965; **46**: 689–97.

14 Katz S, Ford AB, Moskowitz RW *et al.* The Index of ADL: a standardized measure of biological and psychosocial function. *JAMA.* 1963; **185**: 914–19.

15 Lindmark B. Evaluation of functional capacity after stroke with specific emphasis on motor function and ADL. *Scand J Rehabil Med.* 1988; **21S**: 1–40.

16 D'Olhaberriagne L, Litvan I, Panayiotis M *et al.* A reappraisal of reliability and validity studies in stroke. *Stroke.* 1996; **27**: 2331–6.

17 Kasner S. Clinical interpretation and use of stroke scales. *Lancet Neurol.* 2006; **5**: 603–12.

18 Schlegel D, Kolb SJ, Luciano JM *et al.* Utility of the NIH Stroke Scale as a predictor of hospital disposition. *Stroke.* 2003; **34**: 134–7.

## NATIONAL INSTITUTES OF HEALTH STROKE SCALE

This systematic assessment tool was developed in 1983 by NIH-sponsored stroke research neurologists.[1] The National Institutes of Health Stroke Scale (NIHSS) was designed to standardise and document an easy to perform, reliable and valid neurological assessment for use in stroke treatment research trials. Each item was considered with regard to its value during the first few hours and days after symptom onset. This scale is broader than the disability and handicap scales such as the Modified Rankin Scale. It provides a quantitative measure of key components of a standard neurological examination.

### *Scoring*

The NIHSS is a non-linear ordinal scale. The scale has 15 items, and is observer related. The individual items have 3- or 4-point response scales scored from 0 to 3 (where 0 is normal). The total possible score ranges from 0 to 42, with higher scores indicating greater deficit. Subscale items encompass level of consciousness, vision, extra-ocular movements, facial palsy, limb strength, ataxia, sensation, speech and language, and hemineglect. The NIHSS is an observational scale, and measurement by self-report or proxy is not possible.

This scale was designed to be administered in chronological order of items. Because many patients are not as alert at the beginning of the examination as they are at the end, the items that are most difficult to understand are located at the end of the scale. Therefore the scale is administered in chronological order. When scoring, the examiner must score the patient's first attempt. Cuing or coaching should be minimised. Some patients may later correct an error, but changing the score is not permitted. Therefore in general the first response is the most reproducible one. The NIHSS does encourage the use of pantomime and gestures when assessing aphasic or confused patients. Specific pantomime and gesture clues have been developed with the tool to standardise the cuing that may be necessary to score patients. All examiners should score what they actually see, not what they think they should see. Certain items are scored only if they are actually present by examination (e.g. scoring ataxia as '0' or absent in a paralysed or language-impaired patient who cannot move their extremities or comprehend instructions). This approach was taken in order to avoid the use of ambiguous direction, and thereby increase the tool's reproducibility. If the patient is not aphasic but is lethargic or inattentive, alternative assessment techniques may be utilised. The quick and easy reminder form contains cues for the experienced examiner, and the longer teaching version describes all of the examination techniques in more detail (packs available from the National Institute of Neurological Disorders and Stroke Coordinating Centres). Exact clinical findings vary with each possible numerical combination of total score from 0 to 42 (i.e. the total NIHSS score can be the sum total of many possible arithmetical combinations). Therefore caution should be exercised when interpreting the total score.

### Administration time

It takes 5 to 8 minutes to administer the scale.

### Reliability and validity

The NIHSS has established validity and reliability for use in prospective clinical research, and also has predictive validity for long-term stroke outcome.[2] Intra-observer reliability is high, and initial rating followed by re-rating 3 months later yields an inter-class coefficient (ICC) of 0.93,[3] which is near perfect reliability. Inter-observer reliability, with an ICC of 0.95, is also high.[3] The 11-item modified NIHSS (mNIHSS) has 10 items with excellent reliability and 1 item with good reliability.[4] Concurrent validity of the NIHSS has been tested by correlation with infarct volumes using CT or MRI in several studies, yielding correlation coefficients of 0.4–0.8, which suggest a high degree of validity.[5] The clinical predictive validity of the NIHSS has also been demonstrated in several trials.[2,6]

### Clinical application

The NIHSS is a practical and easy-to-use scale. It offers a more expeditious approach, as it can be effectively used by all types of healthcare personnel, whether neurologists or nurses, with excellent reliability and validity after only a few hours' training.[3] The scale then provides a quick and accurate assessment of stroke-related deficits which are easily communicated to other clinicians, thereby saving valuable time in triage and treatment of patients. This is most important when acute thrombolytic treatments must be initiated as soon as possible in order to maximise the benefits ('time is brain'). NIHSS training and certification using a digital video are available and reliable.[7] Training is especially useful in multi-centre trials for standardisation. The NIHSS is currently a key measurement tool in thrombolytic trials.

This scale is also a sensitive tool for serial monitoring of patients following stroke. A change of ≥ 2 points on the NIHSS has been used in trials to suggest a relevant clinical change.[2] Although a specific cut-off value has not been independently validated, a quantifiable change in neurological examination can be quickly recognised and could prompt further diagnostic studies and treatment.[8] Many hospitals have trained nurses to use the NIHSS in bedside monitoring of patients with acute stroke. Online training is available at http://asa.trainingcampus.net

Although the NIHSS is a research tool, it can be easily incorporated into bedside care. Stroke scale checklists can be used to clearly document neurological outcome, to plan safe nursing care and to provide consistency in the informal exchanges between nurses and other healthcare professionals. A nurse's ability to assess and detect early change can have a key role in identifying and affecting the patient outcome in an acutely ill stroke patient.

The NIHSS can aid the planning of a patient's rehabilitation or long-term care needs. The majority of patients with a score of ≤ 5 at the time of admission are likely to be discharged home, those with scores in the range 6–13 usually require inpatient rehabilitation, and those with scores of ≥ 14 frequently need long-term care.[9] Baseline scores strongly predict outcome at 7 days and 3 months, with an excellent outcome in two-thirds of patients with a score of ≤ 3, and very few patients with a score of > 15 having good outcomes.[2]

The NIHSS is a key scale that is useful for clinical research, as it is more sensitive than the Modified Rankin Scale or the Barthel Index in measuring a simulated treatment effect.[10] This is important in clinical research, as greater power for detection of a difference between interventions can allow a smaller sample size.

### Limitations

The NIHSS does not include a detailed assessment of the cranial nerves. Relatively low scores can occur in patients with disabling infarction of brainstem or cerebellum. This scale does not help to identify the actual cause of neurological deficit. Other neurological disorders can mimic stroke, and if an accurate diagnosis is to be obtained, a complete history, neurological examination and neuroimaging are needed. The median volume of right hemispheric strokes and left hemispheric strokes may not correlate for equivalent NIHSS scores. The NIHSS is not an ideal solitary measure for assessing stroke outcomes, and other factors should be taken into account.

Eight-item and 5-item versions of the NIHSS have also been used for pre-hospital screening of patients with suspected stroke.[11]

# NATIONAL INSTITUTES OF HEALTH STROKE SCALE

## N I H STROKE SCALE

Patient Identification. ___ __-___ ___ __-___ ___

Pt. Date of Birth ___ ___/___ ___/___ ___

Hospital _____ (___ -___ )

Date of Exam ___ ___/___ ___/___ ___

Interval: [ ] Baseline  [ ] 2 hours post treatment  [ ] 24 hours post onset of symptoms ±20 minutes  [ ] 7-10 days
[ ] 3 months  [ ] Other _____(___ ___)

Time: ___ ___:___ ___  [ ]am  [ ]pm

Person Administering Scale _____

Administer stroke scale items in the order listed. Record performance in each category after each subscale exam. Do not go back and change scores. Follow directions provided for each exam technique. Scores should reflect what the patient does, not what the clinician thinks the patient can do. The clinician should record answers while administering the exam and work quickly. Except where indicated, the patient should not be coached (i.e., repeated requests to patient to make a special effort).

| Instructions | Scale Definition | Score |
|---|---|---|
| **1a. Level of Consciousness:** The investigator must choose a response if a full evaluation is prevented by such obstacles as an endotracheal tube, language barrier, orotracheal trauma/bandages. A 3 is scored only if the patient makes no movement (other than reflexive posturing) in response to noxious stimulation. | 0 = **Alert**; keenly responsive.<br>1 = **Not alert**; but arousable by minor stimulation to obey, answer, or respond.<br>2 = **Not alert**; requires repeated stimulation to attend, or is obtunded and requires strong or painful stimulation to make movements (not stereotyped).<br>3 = Responds only with reflex motor or autonomic effects or totally unresponsive, flaccid, and areflexic. | _____ |
| **1b. LOC Questions:** The patient is asked the month and his/her age. The answer must be correct - there is no partial credit for being close. Aphasic and stuporous patients who do not comprehend the questions will score 2. Patients unable to speak because of endotracheal intubation, orotracheal trauma, severe dysarthria from any cause, language barrier, or any other problem not secondary to aphasia are given a 1. It is important that only the initial answer be graded and that the examiner not "help" the patient with verbal or non-verbal cues. | 0 = **Answers** both questions correctly.<br>1 = **Answers** one question correctly.<br>2 = **Answers** neither question correctly. | _____ |
| **1c. LOC Commands:** The patient is asked to open and close the eyes and then to grip and release the non-paretic hand. Substitute another one step command if the hands cannot be used. Credit is given if an unequivocal attempt is made but not completed due to weakness. If the patient does not respond to command, the task should be demonstrated to him or her (pantomime), and the result scored (i.e., follows none, one or two commands). Patients with trauma, amputation, or other physical impediments should be given suitable one-step commands. Only the first attempt is scored. | 0 = **Performs** both tasks correctly.<br>1 = **Performs** one task correctly.<br>2 = **Performs** neither task correctly. | _____ |
| **2. Best Gaze:** Only horizontal eye movements will be tested. Voluntary or reflexive (oculocephalic) eye movements will be scored, but caloric testing is not done. If the patient has a conjugate deviation of the eyes that can be overcome by voluntary or reflexive activity, the score will be 1. If a patient has an isolated peripheral nerve paresis (CN III, IV or VI), score a 1. Gaze is testable in all aphasic patients. Patients with ocular trauma, bandages, pre-existing blindness, or other disorder of visual acuity or fields should be tested with reflexive movements, and a choice made by the investigator. Establishing eye contact and then moving about the patient from side to side will occasionally clarify the presence of a partial gaze palsy. | 0 = **Normal.**<br>1 = **Partial gaze palsy;** gaze is abnormal in one or both eyes, but forced deviation or total gaze paresis is not present.<br>2 = **Forced deviation,** or total gaze paresis not overcome by the oculocephalic maneuver. | _____ |

Rev 10/1/2003

# N I H
# STROKE
# SCALE

Patient Identification. ___ ___-___ ___-___ ___ ___

Pt. Date of Birth ___ ___/___ ___/___ ___

Hospital _____ (___ ___-___ ___)

Date of Exam ___ ___/___ ___/___ ___

Interval: [ ] Baseline    [ ] 2 hours post treatment    [ ] 24 hours post onset of symptoms ±20 minutes    [ ] 7-10 days
[ ] 3 months  [ ] Other _____ (___ ___)

| | | |
|---|---|---|
| **3. Visual:** Visual fields (upper and lower quadrants) are tested by confrontation, using finger counting or visual threat, as appropriate. Patients may be encouraged, but if they look at the side of the moving fingers appropriately, this can be scored as normal. If there is unilateral blindness or enucleation, visual fields in the remaining eye are scored.  Score 1 only if a clear-cut asymmetry, including quadrantanopia, is found.  If patient is blind from any cause, score 3. Double simultaneous stimulation is performed at this point.  If there is extinction, patient receives a 1, and the results are used to respond to item 11. | 0 = **No visual loss.**<br><br>1 = **Partial hemianopia.**<br><br>2 = **Complete hemianopia.**<br><br>3 = **Bilateral hemianopia** (blind including cortical blindness). | ____ |
| **4. Facial Palsy:** Ask – or use pantomime to encourage – the patient to show teeth or raise eyebrows and close eyes.  Score symmetry of grimace in response to noxious stimuli in the poorly responsive or non-comprehending patient.  If facial trauma/bandages, orotracheal tube, tape or other physical barriers obscure the face, these should be removed to the extent possible. | 0 = **Normal** symmetrical movements.<br>1 = **Minor paralysis** (flattened nasolabial fold, asymmetry on smiling).<br>2 = **Partial paralysis** (total or near-total paralysis of lower face).<br>3 = **Complete paralysis** of one or both sides (absence of facial movement in the upper and lower face). | ____ |
| **5. Motor Arm:** The limb is placed in the appropriate position: extend the arms (palms down) 90 degrees (if sitting) or 45 degrees (if supine).  Drift is scored if the arm falls before 10 seconds.  The aphasic patient is encouraged using urgency in the voice and pantomime, but not noxious stimulation.  Each limb is tested in turn, beginning with the non-paretic arm.  Only in the case of amputation or joint fusion at the shoulder, the examiner should record the score as untestable (UN), and clearly write the explanation for this choice. | 0 = **No drift;** limb holds 90 (or 45) degrees for full 10 seconds.<br>1 = **Drift;** limb holds 90 (or 45) degrees, but drifts down before full 10 seconds; does not hit bed or other support.<br>2 = **Some effort against gravity;** limb cannot get to or maintain (if cued) 90 (or 45) degrees, drifts down to bed, but has some effort against gravity.<br>3 = **No effort against gravity;** limb falls.<br>4 = **No movement.**<br>UN = **Amputation** or joint fusion, explain: _____<br><br>**5a.  Left Arm**<br><br>**5b.  Right Arm** | <br><br><br>____<br><br>____ |
| **6. Motor Leg:** The limb is placed in the appropriate position: hold the leg at 30 degrees (always tested supine).  Drift is scored if the leg falls before 5 seconds.  The aphasic patient is encouraged using urgency in the voice and pantomime, but not noxious stimulation.  Each limb is tested in turn, beginning with the non-paretic leg.  Only in the case of amputation or joint fusion at the hip, the examiner should record the score as untestable (UN), and clearly write the explanation for this choice. | 0 = **No drift;** leg holds 30-degree position for full 5 seconds.<br>1 = **Drift;** leg falls by the end of the 5-second period but does not hit bed.<br>2 = **Some effort against gravity;** leg falls to bed by 5 seconds, but has some effort against gravity.<br>3 = **No effort against gravity;** leg falls to bed immediately.<br>4 = **No movement.**<br>UN = **Amputation** or joint fusion, explain: _____<br><br>**6a.  Left Leg**<br><br>**6b.  Right Leg** | <br><br>____ |

Rev 10/1/2003

# N I H
# STROKE
# SCALE

Patient Identification. _____ - _____ - _____

Pt. Date of Birth _____ / _____ / _____

Hospital _____ ( _____ - _____ )

Date of Exam _____ / _____ / _____

Interval: [ ] Baseline   [ ] 2 hours post treatment   [ ] 24 hours post onset of symptoms ±20 minutes   [ ] 7-10 days
[ ] 3 months   [ ] Other _____ ( _____ _____ )

| | | |
|---|---|---|
| **7. Limb Ataxia:** This item is aimed at finding evidence of a unilateral cerebellar lesion. Test with eyes open. In case of visual defect, ensure testing is done in intact visual field. The finger-nose-finger and heel-shin tests are performed on both sides, and ataxia is scored only if present out of proportion to weakness. Ataxia is absent in the patient who cannot understand or is paralyzed. Only in the case of amputation or joint fusion, the examiner should record the score as untestable (UN), and clearly write the explanation for this choice. In case of blindness, test by having the patient touch nose from extended arm position. | 0 = **Absent.**<br><br>1 = **Present in one limb.**<br><br>2 = **Present in two limbs.**<br><br>UN = **Amputation** or joint fusion, explain: _____ | _____ |
| **8. Sensory:** Sensation or grimace to pinprick when tested, or withdrawal from noxious stimulus in the obtunded or aphasic patient. Only sensory loss attributed to stroke is scored as abnormal and the examiner should test as many body areas (arms [not hands], legs, trunk, face) as needed to accurately check for hemisensory loss. A score of 2, "severe or total sensory loss," should only be given when a severe or total loss of sensation can be clearly demonstrated. Stuporous and aphasic patients will, therefore, probably score 1 or 0. The patient with brainstem stroke who has bilateral loss of sensation is scored 2. If the patient does not respond and is quadriplegic, score 2. Patients in a coma (item 1a=3) are automatically given a 2 on this item. | 0 = **Normal;** no sensory loss.<br><br>1 = **Mild-to-moderate sensory loss;** patient feels pinprick is less sharp or is dull on the affected side; or there is a loss of superficial pain with pinprick, but patient is aware of being touched.<br><br>2 = **Severe to total sensory loss;** patient is not aware of being touched in the face, arm, and leg. | _____ |
| **9. Best Language:** A great deal of information about comprehension will be obtained during the preceding sections of the examination. For this scale item, the patient is asked to describe what is happening in the attached picture, to name the items on the attached naming sheet and to read from the attached list of sentences. Comprehension is judged from responses here, as well as to all of the commands in the preceding general neurological exam. If visual loss interferes with the tests, ask the patient to identify objects placed in the hand, repeat, and produce speech. The intubated patient should be asked to write. The patient in a coma (item 1a=3) will automatically score 3 on this item. The examiner must choose a score for the patient with stupor or limited cooperation, but a score of 3 should be used only if the patient is mute and follows no one-step commands. | 0 = **No aphasia;** normal.<br><br>1 = **Mild-to-moderate aphasia;** some obvious loss of fluency or facility of comprehension, without significant limitation on ideas expressed or form of expression. Reduction of speech and/or comprehension, however, makes conversation about provided materials difficult or impossible. For example, in conversation about provided materials, examiner can identify picture or naming card content from patient's response.<br><br>2 = **Severe aphasia;** all communication is through fragmentary expression; great need for inference, questioning, and guessing by the listener. Range of information that can be exchanged is limited; listener carries burden of communication. Examiner cannot identify materials provided from patient response.<br><br>3 = **Mute, global aphasia;** no usable speech or auditory comprehension. | _____ |
| **10. Dysarthria:** If patient is thought to be normal, an adequate sample of speech must be obtained by asking patient to read or repeat words from the attached list. If the patient has severe aphasia, the clarity of articulation of spontaneous speech can be rated. Only if the patient is intubated or has other physical barriers to producing speech, the examiner should record the score as untestable (UN), and clearly write an explanation for this choice. Do not tell the patient why he or she is being tested. | 0 = **Normal.**<br>1 = **Mild-to-moderate dysarthria;** patient slurs at least some words and, at worst, can be understood with some difficulty.<br>2 = **Severe dysarthria;** patient's speech is so slurred as to be unintelligible in the absence of or out of proportion to any dysphasia, or is mute/anarthric.<br>UN = **Intubated** or other physical barrier, explain:_____ | _____ |

Rev 10/1/2003

# N I H
# STROKE
# SCALE

Patient Identification. ___ ___-___ ___ ___-___ ___ ___

Pt. Date of Birth ___ / ___ / ___

Hospital _____ (___ -___ ___)

Date of Exam ___ / ___ / ___

Interval: [ ] Baseline    [ ] 2 hours post treatment    [ ] 24 hours post onset of symptoms ±20 minutes    [ ] 7-10 days
[ ] 3 months  [ ] Other _____ (___ ___)

| 11. **Extinction and Inattention (formerly Neglect):** Sufficient information to identify neglect may be obtained during the prior testing. If the patient has a severe visual loss preventing visual double simultaneous stimulation, and the cutaneous stimuli are normal, the score is normal. If the patient has aphasia but does appear to attend to both sides, the score is normal. The presence of visual spatial neglect or anosagnosia may also be taken as evidence of abnormality. Since the abnormality is scored only if present, the item is never untestable. | 0 = **No abnormality.**<br><br>1 = **Visual, tactile, auditory, spatial, or personal inattention** or extinction to bilateral simultaneous stimulation in one of the sensory modalities.<br><br>2 = **Profound hemi-inattention or extinction to more than one modality;** does not recognize own hand or orients to only one side of space. | _____ |

Rev 10/1/2003

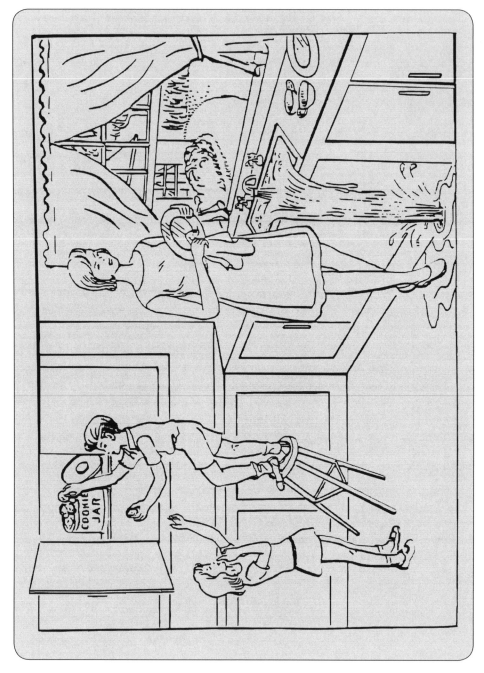

**You know how.**

**Down to earth.**

**I got home from work.**

**Near the table in the dining room.**

**They heard him speak on the radio last night.**

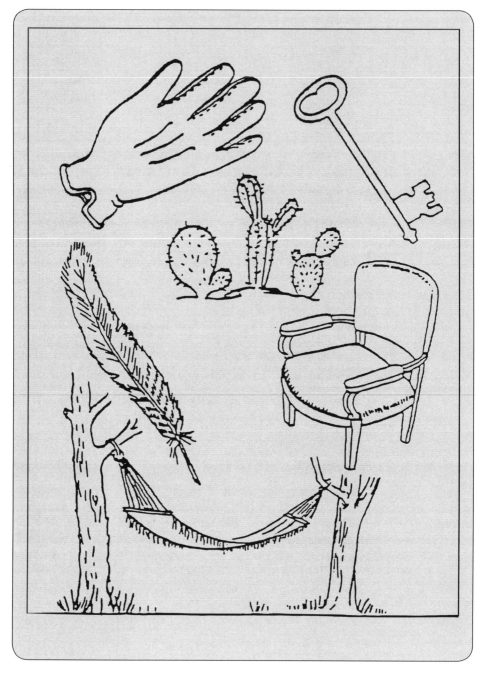

# MAMA

# TIP – TOP

# FIFTY – FIFTY

# THANKS

# HUCKLEBERRY

# BASEBALL PLAYER

Reproduced with the permission of the National Institute of Neurological Disorders and Stroke.

The complete scale can also be obtained from www.ninds.nih.gov/doctors/ NIH_Stroke_Scale.pdf

## REFERENCES

1 Brott T, Adams HP, Olinger CP *et al.* Measurements of acute cerebral infarction: a clinical examination scale. *Stroke.* 1989; **20**: 864–70.

2 Adams HP Jr, Davis PH, Leira EC *et al.* Baseline NIH Stroke Scale strongly predicts outcome after stroke: a report of the Trial of Org 10172 in Acute Stroke Treatment (TOAST). *Neurology.* 1999; **53**: 126–31.

3 Goldstein LB, Samsa GP. Reliability of the National Institutes of Health Stroke Scale: extension to non-neurologists in the context of a clinical trial. *Stroke.* 1997; **28**: 307–10.

4 Meyer BC, Henmen TM, Jackson CM *et al.* Modified National Institutes of Health Stroke Scale for use in stroke clinical trials: prospective reliability and validity. *Stroke.* 2002; **33**: 1261–6.

5 Brott TG, Adams HP Jr, Olinger CP *et al.* Measurements of acute cerebral infarction: a clinical examination scale. *Stroke.* 1989. **20**: 864–70.

6 Schlegel DJ, Tanne D, Demchuk AM *et al.* for the Multicenter rt-PA Stroke Survey Group. Prediction of hospital disposition after thrombolysis for acute ischemic stroke using the National Institutes of Health Stroke Scale. *Arch Neurol.* 2004: **61**: 1061–4.

7 Lyden P, Raman R, Liv L *et al.* NIHSS training and certification using a new digital video disc is reliable. *Stroke.* 2005; **36**: 2446–9.

8 Kasner SE. Clinical interpretation and use of stroke scales. *Lancet Neurol.* 2006; **5**: 603–12.

9 Schegel D, Kolb SJ, Luciano JM *et al.* Utility of the NIH Stroke Scale as a predictor of hospital disposition. *Stroke.* 2003; **34**: 134–7.

10 Young FB, Weir CJ, Lees KR for the GAIN International Trial Steering Committee and Investigators. Comparison of the National Institutes of Health Stroke Scale with disability outcome measures in acute stroke trials. *Stroke.* 2005; **36**: 2187–92.

11 Tirschwell DL, Longstreth WT Jr, Becker KJ *et al.* Shortening the NIH Stroke Scale for use in the prehospital setting. *Stroke.* 2002; **33**: 2801–6.

## GERIATRIC DEPRESSION SCORE

The Geriatric Depression Score (GDS) is used to rate depression in elderly people, and was first introduced in 1983.[1] It is a self-reported inventory with simple 'Yes/No' answers which can be used by the older person or by the interviewer. The GDS can be quickly administered by non-physicians. It is not valid in cognitively impaired people. It is very widely used in old age psychiatry and geriatrics. Several versions are available, ranging from a 30-item version to a 15-item version (the commonest form of the scale) to a 4-item scale.

## GDS-30

This scale is derived from an 100-question scale. During the development of the scale, items were selected from a pool of 100 potential questions to correlate most highly with the total score. This method removed questions about somatic complaints, such as anorexia, weight loss, insomnia and cardiac symptoms.

### Scoring

The GDS-30 is either interviewer- or self-administered. The time frame is the past week. The scale has 30 point-scoring questions with 'Yes/No' answers. Of the 30 items, 20 indicate the presence of depression when answered positively, while 10 items (items 1, 5, 7, 9, 15, 19, 21, 27, 29 and 30) indicate depression when answered negatively. The total score is calculated by totalling 1 point counted for each depression answer:

- score of 0–9: no depression
- score of 10–19: mild depression
- score of 20–30: severe depression.

The answers to the questions are simple, and this instrument does not always require a trained interviewer. The elderly may be reluctant to answer sensitive questions, but this problem can be alleviated by the interviewer providing an explanation.

### Time

It takes 5 to 10 minutes to administer the GDS-30.

### Reliability and validity

This scale has shown 84% sensitivity and 95% specificity at a cut-off value of 11.[2] It has high test–retest reliability and internal consistency. It correlates well with the diagnostic criteria for depression. The GDS-30 is a valid assessment tool for the presence of depression even among institutionalised people with mild to moderate dementia. It has excellent concurrent validity with the Zung Self-Rating Depression Scale and the Hamilton Depression Rating Scale.[3]

### Clinical application

The GDS-30 serves both to screen for depression and as an indicator of the severity of depression. The scale has been used in both hospital and community populations. It performs satisfactorily in the following groups of elderly patients:

- acute medical admissions
- chronic physical illnesses
- specific illnesses (e.g. hip fracture, stroke).

---

**GDS-30**

Patient: ....................... Examiner: ................ Date: ......

Directions to patient: Please choose the best answer for how you have felt over the past week.

Directions to examiner: Present questions *verbally*. Circle the answer given by the patient. Do not show the answer to the patient.

| | | |
|---|---|---|
| 1. Are you basically satisfied with your life? | Yes | **No (1)** |
| 2. Have you dropped many of your activities and interests? | **Yes (1)** | No |
| 3. Do you feel that your life is empty? | **Yes (1)** | No |
| 4. Do you often get bored? | **Yes (1)** | No |
| 5. Are you hopeful about the future? | Yes | **No (1)** |
| 6. Are you bothered by thoughts you can't get out of your head? | **Yes (1)** | No |
| 7. Are you in good spirits most of the time? | Yes | **No (1)** |
| 8. Are you afraid that something bad is going to happen to you? | **Yes (1)** | No |
| 9. Do you feel happy most of the time? | Yes | **No (1)** |
| 10. Do you often feel helpless? | **Yes (1)** | No |
| 11. Do you often get restless and fidgety? | **Yes (1)** | No |
| 12. Do you prefer to stay at home rather than go out and do things? | **Yes (1)** | No |
| 13. Do you frequently worry about the future? | **Yes (1)** | No |
| 14. Do you feel you have more problems with memory than usual? | **Yes (1)** | No |

---

| | | | |
|---|---|---|---|
| 15. | Do you think it is wonderful to be alive now? | Yes | **No (1)** |
| 16. | Do you feel downhearted and blue? | **Yes (1)** | No |
| 17. | Do you feel pretty worthless the way you are now? | **Yes (1)** | No |
| 18. | Do you worry a lot about the past? | **Yes (1)** | No |
| 19. | Do you find life very exciting? | Yes | **No (1)** |
| 20. | Is it hard for you to get started on new projects? | **Yes (1)** | No |
| 21. | Do you feel full of energy? | Yes | **No (1)** |
| 22. | Do you feel that your situation is hopeless? | **Yes (1)** | No |
| 23. | Do you think that most people are better off than you are? | **Yes (1)** | No |
| 24. | Do you frequently get upset over little things? | **Yes (1)** | No |
| 25. | Do you frequently feel like crying? | **Yes (1)** | No |
| 26. | Do you have trouble concentrating? | **Yes (1)** | No |
| 27. | Do you enjoy getting up in the morning? | Yes | **No (1)** |
| 28. | Do you prefer to avoid social occasions? | **Yes (1)** | No |
| 29. | Is it easy for you to make decisions? | Yes | **No (1)** |
| 30. | Is your mind as clear as it used to be? | Yes | **No (1)** |

TOTAL: Please sum all bolded answers (worth one point) for a total score_____

Scores in the range 0–9: normal.

Scores in the range 10–19: mild depression.

Scores in the range 20–30: severe depression.

Reproduced with the permission of the Hartford Institute for Geriatric Nursing, College of Nursing, New York University (personal communication).

Source: www.stanford.edu/~yesavage

## GDS-15

This scale is a 15-item version of the depression scale first described by Sheikh and Yesavage in 1986.[4] It correlates significantly with the 30-point GDS scale. In this scale the somatic symptoms which are less useful as indicators of depression are avoided. Using a cut-off value of 6/7 this scale has similar sensitivity to the parent scale in cognitively intact individuals (78%), but lower specificity (67%). A lower cut-off value of 4/5 gives a specificity of only 48%, but identifies 93% of depressed subjects. This lower cut-off point is useful as a brief screen for depression, and low specificity is acceptable.

The GDS-15 is recommended jointly by the Royal College of Physicians and the British Geriatrics Society as the screening test for depression.

Although different sensitivities and specificities have been obtained across studies, for clinical purposes a score >5 points is suggestive of depression and should warrant a follow-up interview. Scores of >10 are almost always depression.

---

### YESAVAGE GDS–15

Choose the best answer for how you have felt over the past week.

| | | |
|---|---|---|
| 1. | Are you basically happy with your life. | yes/NO |
| 2. | Have you dropped many of your activities and interests. | YES/no |
| 3. | Do you feel that your life is empty. | YES/no |
| 4. | Do you often get bored. | YES/no |
| 5. | Are you in good spirits most of the time. | yes/NO |
| 6. | Are you afraid that something bad is going to happen to you. | YES/no |
| 7. | Do you feel happy most of the time. | yes/NO |
| 8. | Do you often feel helpless. | YES/no |
| 9. | Do you prefer to stay at home rather than going out. | YES/no |
| 10. | Do you feel you have more problems with your memory than most. | YES/no |
| 11. | Do you think it is wonderful to be alive. | yes/NO |
| 12. | Do you feel pretty worthless. | YES/no |
| 13. | Do you feel full of energy. | yes/NO |
| 14. | Do you feel your situation is hopeless. | YES/no |
| 15. | Do you think that most people are better off than you. | YES/no |

Answers indicating depression are shown in capitals. Each answer in capitals scores one point.

Scores in the range 0–4: normal.
Scores in the range 5–10: mild depression.
Scores in the range >11: severe depression.

There is no copyright, as the scale is in the public domain.

The GDS-15 can be obtained at www.stanford.edu/~yesavage/GDS.html

## GDS-10 and GDS-4

These scales have also been used to screen for depression.

### REFERENCES

1 Yesavage JA, Brink TL, Rose TL *et al.* Development and validation of a geriatric depression screening scale: a preliminary report. *J Psychiatr Res.* 1983; **17**: 37–49.

2 Brink T, Yesavage J, Lum O *et al.* Screening tests for geriatric depression. *Clin Gerontol.* 1982; **1**: 37–43.

3 O'Riordan TG, Hayes JP, O'Neil D *et al.* The effect of mild to moderate dementia on the Geriatric Depression Scale and on the General Health Questionnaire. *Age Ageing.* 1990; **19**: 57–61.

4 Sheikh JA, Yesavage JA. Geriatric Depression Scale (GDS): recent findings and development of a shorter version. In: Brink T, editor. *Clinical Gerontology: a guide to assessment and intervention.* New York: Howarth Press; 1986.

## HOSPITAL ANXIETY AND DEPRESSION SCALE

This scale was designed to detect the presence and severity of mood disorder likely to be found in non-psychiatric hospital outpatients.[1] The Hospital Anxiety and Depression (HAD) Scale consists of an Anxiety scale and a separate Depression scale.[1]

### Scoring

The HAD can be either self-administered or interviewer-administered. It is ideal for use in a waiting room. There are 14 items on two subscales, of which 7 items measure anxiety (HADS-A) and 7 items measure depression (HAD-D). Ratings are made on 4-point scales which represent the degree of distress. The replies represent feelings during the past week, where:

0 = none
1 = a little
2 = a lot
3 = unbearably

The items on each of the two subscales are then added. The total possible scores range from 0 to 21 for each scale, with higher scores indicating more distress. Various cut-off points have been quoted.

### Time

It takes about 2 minutes to administer the HAD Scale, and this can therefore easily be done in clinical practice.

### Reliability and validity

This scale has demonstrated good reliability for clinical diagnosis, and good validity. The results have shown good correlations with psychiatric assessments. There are low false-positive and false-negative classification rates, and the scores are not affected by concurrent physical illness.

### Clinical application

The scale is simple to use, and is widely utilised to screen for anxiety and depression. It was originally designed for use with hospital outpatients, and attempts to overcome the bias caused by somatic complaints which feature in other scales. The HAD Scale therefore specifically excludes symptoms such as dizziness and headache which may be attributed to a physical illness. It performs extremely well in measuring both caseness and severity of both anxiety and depression in the general population in primary care, as well as in hospital cohorts.[2] The tool can be used not only for screening but also to chart progress over time. The HAD Scale has been used in a wide variety of patients suffering from chronic conditions such as rheumatoid arthritis, irritable bowel disease, malignancy, early dementia and chronic respiratory diseases.[3] It is popular both in clinical practice and as a research tool.

## Guidelines for use of the HAD Scale

▶ Patients choose one of the four responses for each question.
  A = questions related to anxiety.
  D = questions related to depression.
▶ Responses relate to feelings during the past week.
▶ Respondents are encouraged to give their immediate reaction rather than a carefully considered answer.
▶ The score is given in parentheses before each answer.
▶ Scoring for the Depression and Anxiety scales is done separately.
  0–7 = normal.
  8–10 = borderline abnormal.
  11–21 = abnormal.
▶ A threshold of 8 is suggested as a means of including all possible cases, but a score of ≥ 11 means definite cases.[3]

---

**HOSPITAL ANXIETY AND DEPRESSION SCALE**

A. I feel tense or wound up
   (3) Most of the time
   (2) A lot of the time
   (1) Occasionally
   (0) Not at all

D. I still enjoy the things I used to enjoy
   (0) Definitely as much
   (1) Not quite as much
   (2) Only a little
   (3) Hardly at all

A. I get a frightened feeling as if something awful is about to happen
   (3) Definitely and quite badly
   (2) Yes, but not badly
   (1) A little, but it doesn't worry me
   (0) Not at all

---

D.  I can laugh and see the funny side of things
    (0) As much as I always could
    (1) Not quite so much now.
    (2) Definitely not so much
    (3) Not at all

A.  Worrying thoughts go through my mind
    (3) A great deal of the time
    (2) A lot of the time
    (1) Not too often
    (0) Only occasionally

D.  I feel cheerful
    (3) Not at all
    (2) Not often
    (1) Sometimes
    (0) Most of the time

A.  I can sit at ease and feel relaxed
    (0) Definitely
    (1) Usually
    (2) Not often
    (3) Not at all

D.  I feel as if I am slowed down
    (3) Nearly all the time
    (2) Very often
    (1) Sometimes
    (0) Not at all

A.  I get a frightened feeling like 'butterflies' in the stomach
    (0) Not at all
    (1) Occasionally
    (2) Quite often
    (3) Very often

D.  I have lost interest in my appearance
    (3) Definitely
    (2) I don't take as much care as I should
    (1) I may not take quite as much care
    (0) I take as much care as ever

A. I feel restless as if I have to be on the move
   (3) Very much indeed
   (2) Quite a lot
   (1) Not very much
   (0) Not at all

D. I look forward with enjoyment to things
   (0) As much as I ever did
   (1) Rather less than I used to
   (2) Definitely less than I used to
   (3) Hardly at all

A. I get sudden feelings of panic
   (3) Very often
   (2) Quite often
   (1) Not very often
   (0) Not at all

D. I can enjoy a good book or a radio or TV programme
   (0) Often
   (1) Sometimes
   (2) Not often
   (3) Very seldom

Reproduced with the permission of NFER-Nelson Publishing Ltd (www.nfer-nelson.co.uk) from Zigmond AS, Snaith RP. The Hospital Anxiety and Depression Scale. *Acta Psychiatr Scand.* 1983; **67**: 361–70.

## REFERENCES

1 Zigmond AS, Snaith RP. The Hospital Anxiety and Depression Scale. *Acta Psychiatr Scand.* 1983; **67**: 361–70.

2 Bjelland I, Dahl AA, Hang TT *et al.* The validity of the Hospital Anxiety and Depression Scale: an updated literature review. *J Psychosom Res.* 2002; **52**: 69–77.

3 Carroll BT, Kathol RG, Noyes R *et al.* Screening for depression and anxiety in cancer patients using the Hospital Anxiety and Depression Scale. *J Gen Hosp Psychiatry.* 1993; **15**: 69–74.

## SHORT FORM 36

The Short Form 36 (SF-36) was developed by the Rand Corporation in USA from the Rand Health Batteries, which were experiments of health outcome of adults.[1] It is an abbreviated form of a more detailed instrument, the 108-item Medical Outcomes Survey 1992. These batteries were then used in population surveys. The two main short form versions of the Rand Instruments are known as the Short Form 20 (SF-20) and the Short Form 36 (SF-36).

The SF-36 is a 36-item health status questionnaire, and was first published by Ware and colleagues in 1992.[1] It includes 36 of the 149 items used from original measures. It covers physical health, physiological health, mental health, social health and perceptions of health.

### Scoring

The SF-36 can be self-administered, or alternatively it could be administered by computer or by a trained interviewer either in person or by telephone. Respondents are asked about their health over the past 4 weeks. The scale measures 8 dimensions:

- physical functioning: 10 items
- social functioning: 2 items
- role limitations due to physical problems: 4 items
- role limitations due to emotional problems: 3 items
- mental health: 5 items
- energy: 4 items
- pain: 2 items
- general health perception: 5 items.

Item scores are summed and transformed using a scoring algorithm into a scale ranging from 0% (poor health) to 100% (good health). Recording is required before the scores can be summed.[1]

### Time

It takes 5–10 minutes to administer the scale.

### Validity and reliability

The SF-36 has been shown to have good validity, and is more sensitive than the Nottingham Health Profile. It has good internal consistency and test–retest reliability.

### Clinical application

The SF-36 is increasingly being used to measure health-related quality of life. It can measure positive as well as negative health. The scale has been used in both young[2] and elderly people.[3] It performs well in community surveys of older people,[4] and population norms in many countries have been published.[1] Population norms for the UK have been produced from postal surveys.[5]

### Limitations

The scale has questions which are general in nature and not suitable for assessment of disability. It does not include cognition or instrumental ADL, and has limited coverage of ADL. Its sensitivity may vary between different disease and treatment groups. Response rates depend upon patient-related factors such as age and dependency.[6] In addition, there are conflicting findings with regard to its appropriateness in elderly people.[7] The SF-36 has been criticised for its possible floor effects.[7]

Despite these limitations, the SF-36 has been recommended by several organisations as the generic core for assessing health-related quality of life. It is widely used as a proxy measure of broader health-related quality of life because it is multi-dimensional. It is also used in outcome studies[8] and as a generic core in disease-specific batteries.[7] The SF-36 is now the most frequently used measure of generic health status across the world.

## Modified versions

This scale has been modified to give the SF-36-D, which includes depression items. Brazier and colleagues have modified the SF-36 to make it more appropriate for the UK population.[9] This includes anglicisation of language and alteration of the positioning and coding of one of the social functioning items.

A 12-item version of the SF-36 is also available[10] which contains two dimensions instead of eight, and has been validated for use in older people.[11]

The SF-36 scale cannot be reproduced here. Readers can find the scale on the following websites:

www.sf-36.com

www.qualitymetric.com

## REFERENCES

1 Ware JE, Sherbourne CD. The MOS 36-item short-form health survey (SF-36). I. Conceptual framework and item selection. *Med Care*. 1992; **30**: 473–83.

2 Mahler DA, Mackowisk JI. Evaluation of the short-form 36-item questionnaire to measure health-related quality of life in patients with COPD. *Chest*. 1995; **107**: 1585–9.

3 Bombardier C, Melfi CA, Paul J *et al*. Comparison of a generic and a disease-specific measure of pain and physical function after knee replacement surgery. *Med Care*. 1995; **33 (Suppl. 4)**: AS131–44.

4 Walters SJ, Munro J, Brazier JE. Using the SF-36 with older adults: a cross-sectional community-based survey. *Age Ageing*. 2001; **30**: 337–43.

5 Ruta DA, Garratt AM, Wardlow D *et al*. Developing a valid and reliable measure of health outcome for patients with low back pain. *Spine*. 1994; **19**: 1887–96.

6 McHorney CA, Ware JJ, Raczek AE. The MOS 36-Item Short-Form Health Survey (SF-36). II. Psychometric and clinical tests of validity in measuring physical and mental health constructs. *Med Care*. 1993; **31**: 247–63.

7 McHorney CA. Measuring and monitoring general health status in elderly persons: practical and methodological issues in using the SF-36 Health Survey. *Gerontologist*. 1996; **76**: 571–83.

8 Garratt AM, Ruta DA, Abdalla MI *et al*. The SF-36 health survey questionnaire: an outcome measure suitable for routine use within the NHS? *BMJ*. 1993; **306**: 1440–4.

9 Brazier J, Harper R, Jones NMB *et al*. Validating the SF-36 health survey questionnaire: new outcome measure for primary care. *BMJ*. 1992; **305**: 160–64.

10 Ware JE, Kosinski M, Keller SD. A 12-Item Short-Form Health Survey: construction of scales and preliminary tests of reliability and validity. *Med Care*. 1996; **34**: 220–33.

11 Resnick B, Parker R. Simplified scoring and psychometrics of the revised 12-item short-form health survey. *Outcomes Manag Nurs Pract*. 2001; **5**: 161–6.

## MINI NUTRITIONAL ASSESSMENT

This is a simple, quick and easy test. It includes anthropometric measurement, a dietary questionnaire, and global and subjective assessments (self-perception of health and nutrition). The Mini Nutritional Assessment (MNA) is useful as a screening tool in geriatric assessment, as under-nutrition adversely affects the prognosis of patients both in hospital and in the community.[1] Elderly people are susceptible to under-nutrition, and nutrition can affect the outcome of chronic diseases which are prevalent in the elderly. The prevalence of malnutrition is 5–8% in community-dwelling elderly, and 30–60% in hospital or institutionalised elderly.[1]

### Scoring

The tool consists of 18 questions grouped in four categories:

- anthropometric assessment – height, weight and weight loss
- general assessment – 6 questions related to lifestyle, medication and mobility
- dietary assessment – 8 questions related to number of meals, food and fluid intake, and autonomy of feeding
- subjective assessment – self-perception of health and nutrition.

This instrument distinguishes between three categories of patients:

- adequate nutritional status – MNA ≥ 24
- protein calorie malnutrition – MNA < 17
- at risk of malnutrition – MNA 17–23.5.

### Time

It takes around 10 minutes to administer this instrument.

### Validity and reliability

With this scale the sensitivity is 96%, the specificity is 98% and the positive predictive value is 97%.[2]

### Clinical application

This scale is useful for rapid assessment of the nutritional status of patients in outpatient clinics, hospitals and nursing homes. It also predicts hospital mortality. Thus it is possible to identify people at risk of malnutrition (those with a score in the range 17–23.5) before changes in weight or albumin levels occur. In these individuals, poor nutritional status can easily be corrected by simple nutritional intervention. The scale is reliable and easy to use. Nutritional assessment and intervention in hospital could reduce health costs, as subjects with an MNA score of < 17 stay in hospital longer, with increased costs. The MNA could also identify need for pre-operative nutritional intervention. Elderly patients with a low MNA score living in nursing homes can be identified as needing to receive oral nutritional supplementation, which could help to improve body weight and nutritional status. The MNA has also been useful in both general practice and home care. It has been translated into several languages and validated in many clinics worldwide.[2]

### *Limitations*

The MNA cannot be relied upon individually as a definite diagnostic test for under-nutrition.[3] However, in combination with clinical assessments, a food frequency questionnaire, and selected anthropometric, haematological and biochemical variables, this screening tool can be useful for evaluating the complete nutritional status of elderly patients.[3]

## Modified versions

A shorter version, known as the MNA-SF, when used as a screening tool for malnutrition was found to have high sensitivity in acute medical patients.[4]

The length of the original MNA impedes its use as a screening tool. The MNA has been redesigned, and still contains 18 items, but these are administered in two stages.[5] Stage 1 is a screening questionnaire that uses six key parameters and takes around 3 minutes to administer. The maximum possible score is 14. A score of ≥ 12 indicates satisfactory nutritional status with no need for further assessment. A score of ≤ 11 suggests possible malnutrition, and the need to proceed to the second assessment stage of the MNA. This 6-item MNA is as effective as the 18-item MNA for nutritional screening.[5]

The assessment stage has 12 possible questions with a maximum possible score of 16. Once the assessment stage has been completed, its score is added to the screening score in order to obtain the total assessment score or *Malnutrition Indicator Score*.

For low-risk populations this two-step screening can save time. The full MNA is best used with high-risk or ill elderly patients with a high likelihood of malnutrition.

## MINI NUTRITIONAL ASSESSMENT

Last name: .................... First name: .................... Sex: ...

Date: .......... Age: ...... Weight (kg): ......... Height (cm): .........

Complete the screen by filling in the boxes with the appropriate numbers. Add the numbers in the boxes for the screen. If the score is ≤ 11, continue with the assessment to gain a Malnutrition Indicator Score.

### Screening

A.  Has food intake declined over the past 3 months due to loss of appetite, digestive problems, or chewing or swallowing difficulties?

    a. Severe loss of appetite, 0 points

    b. Moderate loss of appetite, 1 point

    c. No loss of appetite, 2 points

B.  Weight loss during last 3 months

    a. Weight loss greater than 3 kg (6.6 lbs), 0 points

    b. Does not know, 1 point

    c. Weight loss between 1 and 3 kg (between 2.2 and 6.6 lbs), 2 points

    d. No weight loss, 3 points

C.  Mobility

    a. Bed or chair bound, 0 points

    b. Able to get out of bed/chair but does not go out, 1 point

    c. Goes out, 2 points

D.  Has suffered physiological stress or acute disease in the past 3 months

    a. Yes, 0 points

    b. No, 2 points

E.  Neuropsychological problems

    a. Severe dementia or depression, 0 points

    b. Mild dementia, 1 point

    c. No psychological problems, 2 points

*Score*

F.  Body mass index (BMI) (weight in kg/height in m$^2$)

    a.  BMI < 19, 0 points

    b.  BMI 19–20, 1 point

    c.  BMI BMI 21–22, 2 points

    d.  BMI ≥ 23, 3 points

Screening score (maximum score 14 points) _____

≥ 12 points: normal, so not at risk – no need to complete assessment.

≤ 11 points: possible malnutrition – continue assessment.

**Assessment**

G.  Lives independently (not in a nursing home or hospital)    *Score*

    a.  No, 0 points

    b.  Yes, 1 point

H.  Takes more than three prescription drugs per day

    a.  Yes, 0 points

    b.  No, 1 point

I.  Pressure sores or skin ulcers

    a.  Yes, 0 points

    b.  No, 1 point

J.  How many full meals does the patient eat daily?

    a.  1 meal, 0 points

    b.  2 meals, 1 point

    c.  3 meals, 2 points

K.  Selected consumption markers for protein intake

At least one serving of dairy products (milk, cheese, yoghurt) per day?

Yes ☐         No ☐

Two or more servings of legumes or eggs per week?

Yes ☐         No ☐

Meat, fish or poultry every day?

Yes ☐         No ☐

K.  a. If 0 or 1 responses of Yes, 0 points

     b. If 2 responses of Yes, 0.5 points

     c. If 3 responses of Yes, 1 point

L.  Consumes two or more servings of fruit or vegetables per day

    No, 0 points

    Yes, 1 point

M.  How much fluid (water, juice, coffee, tea, milk, etc.) is consumed per day? (1 cup = 8 oz)

    a. Less than 3 cups, 0 points

    b. 3 to 5 cups, 0.5 points

    c. More than 5 cups, 1 point

N.  Mode of feeding

    a. Unable to eat without assistance, 0 points

    b. Self-fed with some difficulty, 1 point

    c. Self-fed without any problem, 2 points

O.  Self-view of nutritional status

    a. Views self as being malnourished, 0 points

    b. Is uncertain of nutritional state, 1 point

    c. Views self as having no nutritional problem, 2 points

P.  In comparison with other people of the same age, how do they consider their health status?

    a. Not as good, 0 points

    b. Does not know, 0.5 points

    c. As good, 1 point

    d. Better, 2 points

Q.  Mid-arm circumference (MAC) in cm

    a. MAC < 21, 0 points

    b. MAC 21–22, 0.5 points

    c. MAC > 22, 1 point

R.  Calf circumference (CC) in cm

    a. CC < 31, 0 points

    b. CC $\geq$ 31, 1 point

Assessment score (maximum score 16 points) _____

Screening score _____

Total assessment score or Malnutrition Indicator Score (maximum score 30 points)

_____

**Malnutrition Indicator Score**
≥ 24 points: well nourished.
17–23.5 points: at risk of malnutrition.
< 17 points: malnourished.

Reproduced with the permission of the Serdi Publishing Company and Nestlé from Guigoz Y, Vallas B, Garry PS. The Mini Nutritional Assessment. In: Vellas BJ, Guigoz Y, Garry PJ, Albarede JL, editors. *Nutrition in the Elderly.* Paris: Serdi; 1994. pp. 15–32.

The Mini Nutritional Assessment can also be found at www.mna-elderly.com

## REFERENCES

1 Guigoz Y, Vallas B, Garry PS. The Mini Nutritional Assessment. In: Vellas BJ, Guigoz Y, Garry PJ, Albarede JL, editors. *Nutrition in the Elderly.* Paris: Serdi; 1994. pp. 15–32.

2 Vellas B, Guigoz Y, Garry PJ *et al.* The Mini Nutritional Assessment (MNA) and its use in grading the nutritional state of elderly patients. *Nutrition.* 1999; **15**: 116–22.

3 Gariballa SE, Sinclair AJ. Diagnosing undernutrition in elderly people. *Rev Clin Gerontol.* 1997; **7**: 367–71.

4 Ranhoff AH, Gjoen AU, Mowe M. Screening for malnutrition in elderly acute medical patients: the usefulness of MNA-SF. *J Nutr Health Aging.* 2005; **9**: 221–5.

5 Rubenstein LZ. Development of a short version of the Mini Nutritional Assessment. In: Vellas B, Garry PJ, Guigoz Y, editors. *Mini Nutritional Assessment (MNA). Research and practice in the elderly. Nestlé Clinical and Performance Nutrition Workshop Series. Volume 1.* Philadelphia, PA: Lippincott-Raven; 1998. pp. 101–11.

## SCALES USED IN PARKINSON'S DISEASE

Many rating scales have been developed for use in Parkinson's disease, based upon the following:

1 signs and symptoms items
2 effect of Parkinson's disease on activities of daily living (ADL)
3 effect of Parkinson's disease on quality of life (QOL).

Examples of scales which have been used in PD include the following:

▶ the Hoehn and Yahr scale
▶ the Unified Parkinson's Disease Rating Scale (UPDRS)
▶ the Webster Scale.

The scales that are used in Parkinson's disease cover many aspects of the impairments, disabilities and handicaps which are associated with the disease. Clinical rating scales are useful as outcome measures in drug studies of Parkinson's disease.

### Hoehn and Yahr scale

This scale[1] correlates with the disease severity in Parkinson's disease. It is a short scale that is easy to use. Its reliability has not been tested. It mixes impairment, disability and handicap.

---

**MODIFIED HOEHN AND YAHR STAGING**

Stage 0   = no signs of disease.
Stage 1   = unilateral disease.
Stage 1.5 = unilateral plus axial involvement.
Stage 2   = bilateral disease, without impairment of balance.
Stage 2.5 = mild bilateral disease, with recovery on pull test.
Stage 3   = mild to moderate bilateral disease, some postural instability, and physically independent.
Stage 4   = severe disability, but still able to walk or stand unassisted.
Stage 5   = wheelchair bound or bedridden unless aided.

Reproduced with the permission of Professor Stanley Fahn, USA (personal communication).

---

The Movement Disorders Society Task Force has prepared a critique for this scale.[2] Its strengths include its wide utilisation and acceptance. Higher stages correlate with neuroimaging studies of dopaminergic loss. High correlations exist between the Hoehn and Yahr scale and some standard scales of motor impairment and disability.[2] The weaknesses of the scale are that it is heavily weighted towards postural instability as the primary index of disease severity. Thus it does not consider impairment/disability due to other motor features of Parkinson's disease. There is no information on non-motor problems. Only the mid ranges (Stages 2 to 4) fulfil the criteria for reliability and validity. Direct clinimetric testing data are limited.[2]

## Unified Parkinson Disease Rating Scale

The Unified Parkinson Disease Rating Scale (UPDRS) is a large scale[3] derived from several other scales. It was developed in an attempt to incorporate elements from existing Parkinson's disease scales in order to provide a means of monitoring Parkinson's disease-related disability and impairment. It has increasingly been used as a 'gold standard' instead of the Hoehn and Yahr Scale.

### Scoring

The scale has four parts:
- Part I: mentation, behaviour and mood.
- Part II: activities of daily living (ADL).
- Part III: motor examination.
- Part IV: complications of therapy.

Thus it is a compound scale which captures multiple aspects of Parkinson's disease. It assesses both motor disability (Part II – ADL) and motor impairment (Part III – motor examination).

### Time

It takes 20–40 minutes to administer this scale. The time can be further shortened by self-administration of the mentation and ADL sections by the patient while they are in the waiting room.

### Reliability and validity

UPDRS scores correlate with the Hoehn and Yahr Scale and the Schwab and England Scale.[4] The UPDRS has shown excellent internal consistency across multiple studies, and retains this consistency across stages of disease severity.[5] Inter-rater reliability is adequate for total scores and motor examination.[4] Among 400 subjects with Parkinson's disease the intra-class correlation coefficients were very high (total score, 0.92; mentation, 0.74; ADL, 0.85; motor examination, 0.90).[6] The UPDRS had adequate face validity and satisfactory construct validity. This scale is sensitive to clinical change.

### Clinical application

The UPDRS achieves a comprehensive assessment in patients with Parkinson's disease with its multi-dimensional approach. It has wide usage and global acceptance, and has been utilised in several multi-centre studies. It has been used in studies of either early, mild Parkinson's disease, moderate but stable disease or late, severe disease and motor fluctuations.[7] A teaching videotape is available that standardises the practical application of the scale and enhances inter-rater reliability.[8] The UPDRS is increasingly used as a 'gold standard' reference scale. The motor examination section has been employed to develop surrogate markers for disease progression using SPECT and PET.[9] US and European regulatory agencies rely on the UPDRS for new drug approvals. Almost all trials of surgical interventions for Parkinson's disease, including intracerebral transplantation and deep brain stimulation, have employed the UPDRS.[10]

### Limitations

The UPDRS is uneven with regard to the type of information that it gathers. For example, Section I is conceptually different from Sections II and III, and Section IV has a mixture of 5-point options and Yes/No ratings that are difficult to analyse together. Most intervention studies for dyskinesias or motor fluctuations rely on other scales. Some items of the motor examination, including speech, facial expression, body bradykinesia, action tremor and rigidity, have relatively poor inter-rater reliability. Bradykinesia-related items are over-represented items by comparison with tremor and postural stability. The allocation of items is not consistent. For example, Part II (ADL) includes a mixture of items. The UPDRS has been used in Caucasians, but has not been examined extensively in other ethnic or racial groups. The coexistence of other diseases, such as diabetes, stroke and arthritis, can confound the evaluation of Parkinson's disease-related disability, and the question of how the UPDRS should accommodate these various issues of comorbidity is not specifically addressed. In addition, several non-motor aspects are not covered, such as anhedonia, anxiety, hypersexuality, sleep disorders, fatigue, dysautonomia and dysregulation, and these could be important clinically.

This scale is mainly used in research studies, and is too long for routine clinical use. It provides a comprehensive assessment in subjects with Parkinson's disease, but it fails to assess cognitive function and bowel and bladder problems.

The Movement Disorder Society Task Force has prepared a critique for the UPDRS.[11] Its strengths include its widespread utilisation, its application across the clinical spectrum of Parkinson's disease, its comprehensive coverage of motor symptoms, and its reliability and validity.[11] Its weaknesses include several ambiguities in the written text, inadequate instructions for raters, and the absence of questions on non-motor aspects of Parkinson's disease.[11]

## Webster Scale

This scale[12] is not used nowadays.

---

### UNIFIED PARKINSON'S DISEASE RATING SCALE

**I. Mentation, behaviour and mood**

**1. Intellectual impairment**

0 = None.

1 = Mild. Consistent forgetfulness with partial recollection of events and no other difficulties.

2 = Moderate memory loss, with disorientation and moderate difficulty in handling complex problems. Mild but definite impairment of function at home, with need for occasional prompting.

3 = Severe memory loss with disorientation with regard to time and often to place. Severe impairment in handling problems.

4 = Severe memory loss with orientation preserved to person only. Unable to make judgements or solve problems. Requires much help with personal care. Cannot be left alone at all.

**2. Thought disorder**

0 = None.

1 = Vivid dreaming.

2 = 'Benign' hallucinations with insight retained.

3 = Occasional to frequent hallucinations or delusions, without insight, which could interfere with daily activities.

4 = Persistent hallucinations, delusions or florid psychosis. Not able to care for self.

**3. Depression**

1 = Periods of sadness or guilt greater than normal, but never sustained for days or weeks.

2 = Sustained depression (1 week or more).

---

3 = Sustained depression with vegetative symptoms (insomnia, anorexia, weight loss, loss of interest).

4 = Sustained depression with vegetative symptoms and suicidal thoughts or intent.

### 4. Motivation/initiative

0 = Normal.

1 = Less assertive than usual; more passive.

2 = Loss of initiative or disinterest in elective (non-routine) activities.

3 = Loss of initiative or disinterest in day-to-day (routine) activities.

4 = Withdrawn, complete loss of motivation.

### II. Activities of daily living (for both 'on' and 'off' motor phenomenon)

### 5. Speech

0 = Normal.

1 = Mildly affected. No difficulty in being understood.

2 = Moderately affected. Sometimes asked to repeat statements.

3 = Severely affected. Frequently asked to repeat statements.

4 = Unintelligible most of the time.

### 6. Salivation

0 = Normal.

1 = Slight but definite excess of saliva in mouth; may have night-time drooling.

2 = Moderately excessive saliva; may have minimal drooling.

3 = Marked excess of saliva with some drooling.

4 = Marked drooling, which requires constant tissue or handkerchief.

### 7. Swallowing

0 = Normal.

1 = Rare choking.

2 = Occasional choking.

3 = Requires soft food.

4 = Requires nasogastric tube or gastrostomy feeding.

### 8. Handwriting

0 = Normal.

1 = Slightly slow or small.

2 = Moderately slow or small; all words are legible.

3 = Severely affected; not all words are legible.

4 = The majority of words are not legible.

### 9. Cutting food and handling utensils

0 = Normal.

1 = Somewhat slow and clumsy, but no help is needed.

2 = Can cut most foods, although clumsy and slow; some help is needed.

3 = Food must be cut by someone else, but can still feed slowly.

4 = Needs to be fed.

### 10. Dressing

0 = Normal.

1 = Somewhat slow, but no help is needed.

2 = Occasional assistance with buttoning, and with getting arms into sleeves.

3 = Considerable help required, but can do some things alone.

4 = Helpless.

### 11. Hygiene

0 = Normal.

1 = Somewhat slow, but no help is needed.

2 = Needs help to shower or bathe, or very slow in hygienic care.

3 = Requires assistance with washing, brushing teeth, combing hair, and going to bathroom.

4 = Foley catheter or other mechanical aids.

### 12. Turning in bed and adjusting bedclothes

0 = Normal.

1 = Somewhat slow and clumsy, but no help is needed.

2 = Can turn alone or adjust sheets, but with great difficulty.

3 = Can initiate, but not turn or adjust sheets alone.

4 = Helpless.

### 13. Falling (unrelated to freezing)

0 = None.
1 = Falls rarely.
2 = Falls occasionally, less than once per day.
3 = Falls an average of once daily.
4 = Falls more than once daily.

### 14. Freezing when walking

0 = None.
1 = Rare freezing when walking; may have start hesitation.
2 = Occasional freezing when walking.
3 = Frequent freezing. Occasionally falls from freezing.
4 = Frequent falls from freezing.

### 15. Walking

0 = Normal.
1 = Mild difficulty. May not swing arms or may tend to drag leg.
2 = Moderate difficulty, but requires little or no assistance.
3 = Severe disturbance of walking, requiring assistance.
4 = Cannot walk at all, even with assistance.

### 16. Tremor (symptomatic complaint of tremor in any part of the body)

0 = Absent.
1 = Slight. Infrequently present.
2 = Moderate. Bothersome to patient.
3 = Severe. Interferes with many activities.
4 = Marked. Interferes with most activities.

### 17. Sensory complaints related to parkinsonism

0 = None.
1 = Occasionally has numbness, tingling or mild aching.
2 = Frequently has numbness, tingling or aching; not distressing.
3 = Frequent painful sensations.
4 = Excruciating pain.

### III. Motor examination

### 18. Speech

0 = Normal.
1 = Slight loss of expression, diction and/or volume.

2 = Monotone, slurred but understandable; moderately impaired.

3 = Marked impairment, difficult to understand.

4 = Unintelligible.

### 19. Facial expression

0 = Normal.

1 = Minimal hypomimia, could be normal 'poker face.'

2 = Slight but definitely abnormal diminution of facial expression.

3 = Moderate hypomimia; lips parted some of the time.

4 = Masked or fixed facies with severe or complete loss of facial expression; lips parted a quarter of an inch or more.

### 20. Tremor at rest (head, upper and lower extremities)

0 = Absent.

1 = Slight and infrequently present.

2 = Mild in amplitude and persistent. Or moderate in amplitude, but only intermittently present.

3 = Moderate in amplitude and present most of the time.

4 = Marked in amplitude and present most of the time.

### 21. Action or postural tremor of hands

0 = Absent.

1 = Slight, and present with action.

2 = Moderate in amplitude, and present with action.

3 = Moderate in amplitude with posture holding as well as action.

4 = Marked in amplitude; interferes with feeding.

### 22. Rigidity (judged on passive movement of major joints with patient relaxed in sitting position; cogwheeling to be ignored)

0 = Absent.

1 = Slight or detectable only when activated by mirror or other movements.

2 = Mild to moderate.

3 = Marked, but full range of motion easily achieved.

4 = Severe; range of motion achieved with difficulty.

### 23. Finger taps (patient taps thumb with index finger in rapid succession)

0 = Normal.

1 = Mild slowing and/or reduction in amplitude.

2 = Moderately impaired. Definite and early fatiguing. May have occasional arrests in movement.

3 = Severely impaired. Frequent hesitation in initiating movements or arrests in ongoing movement.

4 = Can barely perform the task.

**24. Hand movements** (patient opens and closes hands in rapid succession)

0 = Normal.

1 = Mild slowing and/or reduction in amplitude.

2 = Moderately impaired. Definite and early fatiguing. May have occasional arrests in movement.

3 = Severely impaired. Frequent hesitation in initiating movements or arrests in ongoing movement.

4 = Can barely perform the task.

**25. Rapid alternating movements of hands** (pronation–supination movements of hands, vertically and horizontally, with as large an amplitude as possible, with both hands simultaneously)

0 = Normal.

1 = Mild slowing and/or reduction in amplitude.

2 = Moderately impaired. Definite and early fatiguing. May have occasional arrests in movement.

3 = Severely impaired. Frequent hesitation in initiating movements or arrests in ongoing movement.

4 = Can barely perform the task.

**26. Leg agility** (patient taps heel on the ground in rapid succession picking up entire leg. Amplitude should be at least 3 inches)

0 = Normal.

1 = Mild slowing and/or reduction in amplitude.

2 = Moderately impaired. Definite and early fatiguing. May have occasional arrests in movement.

3 = Severely impaired. Frequent hesitation in initiating movements or arrests in ongoing movement.

4 = Can barely perform the task.

**27. Arising from chair** (patient attempts to rise from a straight-backed chair, with arms folded across chest)

0 = Normal.

1 = Slow, or may need more than one attempt.

2 = Pushes self up from arms of seat.

3 = Tends to fall back and may have to try more than once, but can get up without help.

4 = Unable to arise without help.

### 28. Posture

0 = Normal erect.

1 = Not quite erect, slightly stooped posture; could be normal for older person.

2 = Moderately stooped posture, definitely abnormal; can be slightly leaning to one side.

3 = Severely stooped posture with kyphosis; can be moderately leaning to one side.

4 = Marked flexion with extreme abnormality of posture.

### 29. Gait

0 = Normal.

1 = Walks slowly, may shuffle with short steps, but no festination (hastening steps) or propulsion.

2 = Walks with difficulty, but requires little or no assistance; may have some festination, short steps or propulsion.

3 = Severe disturbance of gait, requiring assistance.

4 = Cannot walk at all, even with assistance.

### 30. Postural stability (response to sudden, strong posterior displacement produced by pull on shoulders while patient is erect with eyes open and feet slightly apart. Patient is prepared)

0 = Normal.

1 = Retropulsion, but recovers unaided.

2 = Absence of postural response; would fall if not caught by examiner.

3 = Very unstable; tends to lose balance spontaneously.

4 = Unable to stand without assistance.

### 31. Body bradykinesia and hypokinesia (combining slowness, hesitancy, decreased armswing, small amplitude, and poverty of movement in general)

0 = None.

1 = Minimal slowness, giving movement a deliberate character; could be normal for some individuals. Possibly reduced amplitude.

2 = Mild degree of slowness and poverty of movement which is definitely abnormal. Alternatively, some reduced amplitude.

3 = Moderate slowness, poverty or small amplitude of movement.

4 = Marked slowness, poverty or small amplitude of movement.

## IV. Complications of therapy (in the past week)
## A. Dyskinesias
**32. Duration: For what proportion of the waking day are dyskinesias present?**
(historical information)
0 = None
1 = 1–25% of day.
2 = 26–50% of day.
3 = 51–75% of day.
4 = 76–100% of day.

**33. Disability: How disabling are the dyskinesias?** (historical information; may be modified by office examination)
0 = Not disabling.
1 = Mildly disabling.
2 = Moderately disabling.
3 = Severely disabling.
4 = Completely disabled.

**34. Painful dyskinesias: How painful are the dyskinesias?**
0 = No painful dyskinesias.
1 = Slight.
2 = Moderate.
3 = Severe.
4 = Marked.

**35. Presence of early-morning dystonia** (historical information)
0 = No.
1 = Yes.

## B. Clinical fluctuations
**36. Are 'off' periods predictable?**
0 = No.
1 = Yes.

**37. Are 'off' periods unpredictable?**
0 = No.
1 = Yes.

**38. Do 'off' periods come on suddenly, within a few seconds?**
0 = No.
1 = Yes.

**39. For what proportion of the waking day is the patient 'off' on average?**
0 = None.
1 = 1–25% of day.
2 = 26–50% of day.
3 = 51–75% of day.
4 = 76–100% of day.

**C. Other complications**
**40. Does the patient have anorexia, nausea or vomiting?**
0 = No.
1 = Yes.

**41. Does the patient have any sleep disturbances, such as insomnia or hypersomnolence?**
0 = No.
1 = Yes.

**42. Does the patient have symptomatic orthostasis?** (Record the patient's blood pressure, height and weight on the scoring form)
0 = No.
1 = Yes.

Reproduced with the permission of Professor S Fahn (personal communication) from Fahn S, Elton RL. Members of the UPDRS Development Committee. Unified Parkinson's disease rating scale. In: Fahn S, Marsden CD, Calne DB, Goldstein M, editors. *Recent Developments in Parkinson's Disease. Volume 2.* Florham Park, NJ: Macmillan Health Care Information; 1987. pp. 153–64.

## REFERENCES

1 Hoehn MM, Yahr MD. Parkinsonism: onset, progression and mortality. *Neurology.* 1967; **17**: 427–42.
2 Goetz CG, Poewe W, Rascol O *et al.* Movement Disorder Society Task Force report on the Hoehn and Yahr staging scale: status and recommendations. *Mov Disord.* 2004; **19**: 1020–28.

3 Fahn S, Elton RL. Members of the UPDRS Development Committee. Unified Parkinson's disease rating scale. In: Fahn S, Marsden CD, Calne DB, Goldstein M, editors. *Recent Developments in Parkinson's Disease. Volume 2.* Florham Park, NJ: Macmillan Health Care Information; 1987. pp. 153–64.

4 Martinez-Martin P, Gil-Nagel A, Gracia LM *et al.* Unified Parkinson's disease rating scale characteristics and structure. The Co-operative Multicentric Group. *Mov Disord.* 1994; **9**: 76–83.

5 Van Hilten JJ, van der Zwan AD, Zwinderman AH *et al.* Rating impairment and disability in Parkinson's disease: evaluation of the Unified Parkinson's Disease Rating Scale. *Mov Disord.* 1994; **9**: 84–8.

6 Siderowf A, McDermott M, Kieburtz K *et al.* Test–retest reliability of the Unified Parkinson's Disease Rating Scale in patients with early Parkinson's disease: results from a multicenter clinical trial. *Mov Disord.* 2002; **17**: 758–63.

7 Mitchell SL, Harper DW, Bhalla R. Patterns of outcome measurement in Parkinson's disease clinical trials. *Neuroepidemiology.* 2000; **19**: 100–8.

8 Goetz CG, Stebbins GT, Chmura TA *et al.* Teaching tape for the motor section of the Unified Parkinson's Disease Rating Scale. *Mov Disord.* 1995; **10**: 263–6.

9 Morrish PK, Sawle GV, Brooks DJ. An [$^{18}$F]dopa–PET and clinical study of the rate of progression in Parkinson's disease. *Brain.* 1996; **119**: 585–91.

10 Defer GL, Widner H, Marie RM *et al.* Core assessment program for surgical interventional therapies in Parkinson's disease (CAPSIT-PD). *Mov Disord.* 1999; **14**: 572–84.

11 Movement Disorder Society Task Force on Rating Scales for Parkinson's Disease. The Unified Parkinson's Disease Rating Scale (UPDRS): status and recommendations. *Mov Disord.* 2003; **18**: 738–50.

12 Webster DD. Clinical analysis of the disability in Parkinson's disease. *Mod Treat.* 1968; **5**: 257–82

## SCALES USED IN PRESSURE SORE ASSESSMENT

Approximately 9% of all patients admitted to a hospital develop pressure ulcers (pressure sores). Individuals over 65 years of age are at greatest risk. Patients who are at risk of developing pressure sores must be identified and prevention measures undertaken. Proper identification of risk can prevent pressure damage. Numerous risk assessment scales have been devised to assist in the identification of patients who are at risk. Each item is given a numerical value, and the sum of scores represents the total risk score. A threshold score is used to classify patients as either 'at risk' or 'not at risk.' The overall risk score could also be used to guide selection of a mattress or special bed, or when recommending a position-changing regimen. The scales can aid clinical judgement and function as an aide-memoire for less experienced staff. Nowadays, there is an increased emphasis on nurses' accountability, which highlights the need for such scales to assist judgement. The scales are also useful when communicating care planning to colleagues.

The following three standardised scales have been in common usage:

1 the Norton Scale, published in 1962[1]
2 the Waterlow Scale, published in 1985[2]
3 the Pressure Sore Prediction Score, published in 1987.[3]

Comparison of these three scales is difficult. The relative sensitivity and specificity have been used to judge which scale is more closely associated with presence or absence of sores. A highly sensitive scale would identify everyone at risk, and a highly specific scale would detect all those not at risk. If both sensitivity and specificity are high, the scale would be useful for targeting equipment and interventions when needed. In practice the relationship tends to be inverse, such that the higher the sensitivity, the lower the specificity. Moreover, scales that are useful in one setting may not be suitable in another, as each clinical area has specific factors that affect pressure sore development.

The Norton Scale was the earliest to be developed. It was designed for use in Care of the Elderly units,[1] and is not in use now. The Waterlow Scale[2] was developed following two pressure sore surveys by Somerset Health Authority. It has been criticised for over- or under-predicting pressure sore risk.[4] This scale does not display high levels of reliability, and it lacks operational definitions within risk categories.

### Pressure Sore Prediction Score (PSPS)

This scale was devised and published by Lowthian.[3] It was developed at the Royal

National Orthopaedic Hospital in a population of patients with orthopaedic trauma and spinal injuries.

### Scoring

The scale contains six questions about the patient's condition (sitting up, unconscious, poor general condition, incontinent, lifts up, and gets up and walks). The intermediate answers 'Yes but' and 'Yes and no' allow the nurse rater to score indefinite answers to the key questions, and in practice this system is quickly understood even by inexperienced nurses. A score of $\geq 6$ indicates risk of development of pressure ulcers.

## Explanatory notes

▶ These are questions to ask yourself about the patient.
▶ All of the questions concern the patient's state at the time when the scale was completed.
▶ A score of > 6 indicates that the patient is at risk.
▶ If a pressure sore is present, the minimum score is 10.

**PRESSURE SORE PREDICTION SCORE**

|  | No | No but | Yes but | Yes |
|---|---|---|---|---|
| Sitting up? | 0 | 1 | 2 | 3 |
| Unconscious? | 0 | 1 | 2 | 3 |
| Poor general condition? | 0 | 1 | 2 | 3 |
| Incontinent? | 0 | 1 | 2 | 3 |

|  | No | Yes and no | Yes |
|---|---|---|---|
| Lifts up? | 2 | 1 | 0 |
| Gets up and walks? | 2 | 1 | 0 |

Reproduced with the permission of Mcmillan-Scott (originally TVS Publications) from Lowthian P. The practical assessment of pressure sore risk. *Care Sci Pract.* 1987; **5:** 3–7.

### Reliability and validity

This scale has high sensitivity and specificity relative to other published scales.[5] It also has good inter-rater reliability. A validation study has demonstrated a sensitivity of 89% and a specificity of 76%.[6]

## Clinical application

The scale is easy to use, even by untrained staff or in a situation where medical details such as those required by the Waterlow Scale are unavailable. It has been designed to be used by all grades of nurses and in all nursing situations. It is quick and easy to remember, and is in common usage across hospitals in the UK. A recent review demonstrated that it is an effective tool in orthopaedic settings in the UK.[7]

## Limitations

Pressure Sore Prediction Score items include the well-documented risk factors, such as incontinence and level of consciousness. However, the risk factor 'nutrition', which also affects individuals' susceptibility to pressure sore development, is not included.

### REFERENCES

1 Norton D, McLaren R, Exton-Smith AN. *An Investigation of Geriatric Nursing Problems in Hospitals.* London: National Corporation for the Care of Older People; 1962.

2 Waterlow J. A risk assessment card. *Nurs Times.* 1985; **81**: 49–55.

3 Lowthian P. The practical assessment of pressure sore risk. *Care Sci Pract.* 1987; **5**: 3–7.

4 Edwards M. The levels of reliability and validity of the Waterlow pressure sore risk calculator. *J Wound Care.* 1995; **4**: 373–8.

5 Maylor M, Roberts A. A comparison of three risk assessment scales. *Prof Nurse.* 1999; **14**: 629–32.

6 Lowthian P. Identifying and protecting patients who may get pressure sores. *Nurs Standard.* 1989; **4**: 26–9.

7 Mitchell H. A review of the Lowthian pressure sore prediction score for risk assessment in the orthopaedic setting. *J Orthop Nurs.* 2004; **8**: 142–50.

# Conclusion

Frail elderly people have an extensive list of problems. A comprehensive assessment has a clear role in promoting better healthcare. Adequate assessment must be regarded as a prerequisite for appropriate care of elderly people, and is one of the linchpin frameworks of operation and principles of geriatric medicine. Assessment defines the state of physical, mental and social well-being of an individual, and also the needs for services.

A range of assessment scales have been developed to cover a wide range of areas relevant to elderly people. Some are useful in everyday practice, while others are used in research settings. All of the available measurement scales have both strengths and limitations. Those professionals who provide care for elderly people find these scales useful in their daily practice. In order to plan care, practitioners need to measure health and well-being. Measurement scales help to monitor change in health status and thereby assess outcomes. Managers in health and social care need information from such scales to enable them to plan service management. Researchers study these scales to increase their understanding of their properties. The choice of a particular scale is strongly determined by the context of use, in terms of both the purpose of the scale and the characteristics of the population on which it will be used. Instruments that are appropriate in one setting may not be useful in another. In all circumstances the instrument must be valid and reliable. An instrument that is used as an outcome measure must be responsive. Assessment tools can improve practitioners' knowledge about their elderly patients, aid decision making and improve communication both across the multi-disciplinary team and across sectors (hospital and community). Assessment tools can enhance the quality of care. However, it is important that assessment methods in daily practice make life simpler and not more complicated for practitioners and managers in hospital and community care. The additional costs in terms of staff time and the processing of information need to be minimal. Monitoring, audit and evaluation of assessment scales, and also research into these scales, must be ongoing in order to ensure that high-quality care is delivered to elderly people. Many aspects of feasibility, interpretability and usefulness of measurement scales have yet to be established. Future research could help to determine the usefulness of scales in enhancing patient care and thereby improving clinical outcomes.

# Appendix

## SURVEY OF BRITISH GERIATRICS SOCIETY MEMBERS

A study was conducted by myself and Professor Bhowmick by sending a postal questionnaire to 2000 members of the British Geriatrics Society. Responses were received from 149 consultants, 37 specialist registrars and 23 others (staff grades and associate specialists). Even though the response rate was poor, the results indicate that there is wide variation in the familiarity of specialists in geriatric medicine with measurement scales. Very few measurement scales were familiar to and utilised by specialist clinicians working in the UK. It is clear that much more education, training and research is needed to promote familiarity with and consistency of usage of these scales in Elderly Care Units across the UK.

### Response from 149 consultants

| Scale | Familiar with | Frequently use |
|---|---|---|
| GCS | 148 | 128 |
| AMT | 148 | 128 |
| MMSE | 149 | 132 |
| Clock Drawing Test | 138 | 64 |
| CAPE | 49 | 4 |
| Barthel Index | 149 | 95 |
| NEADL | 58 | 3 |
| mRS | 91 | 21 |
| FIM and FAM | 37 | 4 |
| Timed Walking Test | 120 | 43 |
| NIHSS | 67 | 14 |
| GDS-15 | 129 | 76 |
| GDS-30 | 87 | 21 |
| HAD | 96 | 26 |
| SF-36 | 72 | 2 |

| Scale | Familiar with | Frequently use |
|---|---|---|
| MNA | 48 | 11 |
| UPDRS | 87 | 21 |
| Hoehn and Yahr Scale | 82 | 20 |
| PSPS | 90 | 43 |

## Other scales mentioned by consultants

- Waterlow Scale (8 responses).
- Falls Risk STRATIFY.
- BASDEC (2 responses).
- AD BEHAVE.
- Bristol ADL (2 responses).
- Carer Stress Scale.
- LINDOP Parkinson Disease Assessment Scale.
- Berg Balance Scale (3 responses).
- Up and Go Test (2 responses).
- Maelor Sore Prevention Scale.
- Addenbrookes Cognitive Examination.
- Frontal Assessment Battery (2 responses).
- AMT-4.
- CURB Score.
- Wells Score.
- MEWS Rockhall Score.
- Elder Abuse Screening Questionnaire.
- Philadelphia IADL.
- CAGE/FAST 2.
- Neuropsychiatric Inventory.
- Tinneti Balance Scale (2 responses).
- Confusion Assessment Method (2 responses).
- Elderly Mobility Score (3 responses).
- Epworth Sleep scale (3 responses).
- Bamford Stroke Classification.
- Blessed Dementia Rating Scale.
- IQCDE– Informant Questionnaire on Cognitive Decline in the Elderly (2 responses).
- GDS-10.
- GDS-4.
- Hatchinski Scale.
- Hamilton Depression Scale.
- Beck Depression Scale.

- Parkinson's Disease Questionnaire.
- 6CIT (6-item Cognitive Impairment Test).
- CAMCOG.
- TUSS.
- TUAG.
- FRASE (Falls Risk Assessment).
- Instrumental ADL.
- Zaggo's Line Cancellation.
- Isaacs's Set Test.
- Instrumental ADL.
- EQOL.
- ADDQOL.
- Tremor Rigidity and Bradykinesia Score.
- ACE-R.
- Middlesex Elderly Assessment of Mental State.
- Wimbledon Scale.
- CAM4 Tool.
- Oxford Handicap Scale.

## Responses from 37 specialist registrars

| Scale | Familiar with | Frequently use |
| --- | --- | --- |
| GCS | 37 | 36 |
| AMT | 37 | 36 |
| MMSE | 37 | 35 |
| Clock Drawing Test | 34 | 15 |
| CAPE | 3 | 0 |
| Barthel Index | 36 | 20 |
| NEADL | 11 | 0 |
| mRS | 16 | 4 |
| FIM and FAM | 7 | 0 |
| Timed Walking Test | 29 | 11 |
| NIHSS | 22 | 9 |
| GDS-15 | 33 | 15 |
| GDS-30 | 21 | 3 |
| HAD | 26 | 6 |
| SF-36 | 18 | 1 |
| MNA | 14 | 1 |

| Scale | Familiar with | Frequently use |
|---|---|---|
| UPDRS | 22 | 5 |
| Hoehn and Yahr Scale | 20 | 3 |
| PSPS | 14 | 2 |

## Other scales mentioned by specialist registrars

▶ STRATIFY Score.
▶ EUROQOL.
▶ EQ5D.
▶ MUST Score.
▶ Stroke Impact Scale.
▶ Scandinavian Stroke Scale.
▶ CAMS.
▶ Waterlow Scale.
▶ TPP Orientation-3.
▶ CAM-3.
▶ Addenbrookes-100.
▶ Canard.
▶ CURB65 (for pneumonia).
▶ Dundee Functional Outcome Measure.
▶ Hamilton Depression Rating Scale.
▶ MDRS.
▶ Beck DS.
▶ Confusion Assessment Method.
▶ Tinetti Gait and Balance Scale.

## Responses from 23 others (staff grades/associate specialists)

| Scale | Familiar with | Frequently use |
|---|---|---|
| GCS | 21 | 12 |
| AMT | 22 | 17 |
| MMSE | 22 | 18 |
| Clock Drawing Test | 21 | 5 |
| CAPE | 6 | 0 |
| Barthel Index | 22 | 14 |
| NEADL | 3 | 0 |
| mRS | 3 | 1 |
| FIM and FAM | 4 | 1 |
| Timed Walking Test | 19 | 7 |

| Scale | Familiar with | Frequently use |
|-------|:-------------:|:--------------:|
| NIHSS | 4 | 1 |
| GDS-15 | 18 | 14 |
| GDS-30 | 11 | 1 |
| HAD | 15 | 4 |
| SF-36 | 8 | 0 |
| MNA | 2 | 1 |
| UPDRS | 13 | 5 |
| Hoehn and Yahr Scale | 9 | 3 |
| PSPS | 12 | 2 |

## Other scales mentioned by 'others'

▶ Waterlow Scale.
▶ Neuropathic Pain Score.
▶ Webster Score.
▶ Berg Balance Scale.
▶ Elderly Mobility Scale.
▶ Kings Health Questionnaire.
▶ ICI-OAB.
▶ BSAQ.
▶ CAM.
▶ Abbreviated GDS.
▶ Signs of Depression Screening Scale.
▶ Bristol ADL.
▶ Urinary Incontinence QOL Scale.

# Further reading

Royal College of Physicians of London and the British Geriatrics Society. *Standardised Assessment Scales for Elderly People. Report of joint workshops of the Research Unit of Royal College of Physicians of London and the British Geriatrics Society.* London: Royal College of Physicians of London; 1992.

Philp I. *Assessing Elderly People in Hospital and Community Care.* London: Farrand Press; 1994.

Wade DT. *Measurement in Neurological Rehabilitation.* Oxford: Oxford Medical Publications; 1992.

McDowell I. *Measuring Health: a guide to rating scales and questionnaires.* 3rd ed. Oxford: Oxford University Press; 2006.

Kane RL, Kane RA. *Assessing Older Persons: measures, meaning and practical applications.* Oxford: Oxford University Press; 2000.

Streiner DL, Norman GR. *Health Measurement Scales. A practical guide to their development and use.* 3rd ed. Oxford: Oxford Medical Publications; 2003.

Corcoran K, Fischer J. *Measures for Clinical Practice: a sourcebook.* New York: Free Press; 1987.

Bowling A. *Measuring Health: a review of quality of life measurement scales.* 3rd ed. Buckingham: Open University Press; 2005.

Bowling A. *Measuring Disease: a review of disease-specific quality of life measurement scales.* 2nd ed. Buckingham: Open University Press; 2001.

Bolton B. Measurement in rehabilitation. In: Pan EL, Newman SS, Backer TE *et al.*, editors. *Annual Review of Rehabilitation. Volume 4.* New York: Springer; 1985.

Wilkin D, Hallam L, Doggett MA. *Measures of Need and Outcome for Primary Health Care.* Oxford: Oxford University Press; 1992.

Rubenstein LZ, Wieland D, Bernabei R. *Geriatric Assessment: the state of the art.* Milan: Editrice Kurtis; 1995.

Kane RA, Kane RL. *Assessing the Elderly: a practical guide to measurement.* Toronto: Lexington Books; 1981.

Shumway Cook A, Woolacott MH. *Motor Control: theory and practical applications.* Philadelphia, PA: Lippincott, Williams and Wilkins; 2001.

# Index